FIBER DEFICIENCY AND COLONIC DISORDERS

FIBER DEFICIENCY AND COLONIC DISORDERS

Edited by

Richard W. Reilly
and
Joseph B. Kirsner

Department of Medicine
The Pritzker School of Medicine
The University of Chicago

PLENUM MEDICAL BOOK COMPANY • New York and London

Library of Congress Cataloging in Publication Data

Main entry under title:

Fiber deficiency and colonic disorders.

"Invited papers presented at a conference held in the Center for Continuing Educa-
tion, University of Chicago, under the sponsorship of the Gastroenterology Section
of the Department of Medicine at the university, on May 17, 1974."
Includes bibliographies and index.
1. High-fiber diet—Congresses. 2. Colon (Anatomy)—Diseases—Congresses. I. Reilly,
Richard W. II. Kirsner, Joseph Barnett, 1909-   III. Pritzker School of Medicine.
Dept. of Medicine. Gastroenterology Section. [DNLM: 1. Colonic diseases—Etiology—
Congresses. 2. Cellulose—Deficiency—Congresses. QU75 F443 1974]

RM237.6.F52	616.3'4	75-12756

ISBN-13: 978-1-4684-2174-3   e-ISBN-13: 978-1-4684-2172-9
DOI: 10.1007/978-1-4684-2172-9

Invited papers presented at a conference held in
The Center for Continuing Education, University of Chicago,
under the sponsorship of the Gastroenterology Section of
the Department of Medicine at the University, on May 17, 1974

Foreword

Epidemiologists, on the basis of studies carried out chiefly in Africa, have suggested that depletion of fiber in the modern Western diet affects health adversely. D. P. Burkitt, who has been in the forefront of this investigation, has included among the "diseases of civilization" hiatus hernia, ischemic heart disease, cholelithiasis, polyps of the colon, and cancer of the colon. All of these conditions appear to have the same geographic distribution. In these areas, the diets were characterized by increased amounts of fat and meat protein, and by an apparent deficit of fiber. It is noteworthy that while an increased intake of refined sugars also has been implicated in the Western diet, the consumption of sugar and other sweetners in the United States actually has remained fairly stable since about 1925 when the use of complex carbohydrates in the form of starchy foods began to decline. The mechanism whereby deficiency of fiber in the diet contributes to the development of colonic diverticula, presumably is by facilitating the development of segmentation of the colon and pockets of intracolonic high pressure zones associated with prolonged transit time of bowel content. Preliminary therapeutic observations, furthermore, have suggested that the addition of fiber in the form of bran to the diet may promote regularity of bowel function and perhaps lessen the likelihood that new diverticula will be formed after the resection of involved colonic segments. In relation to the pathogenesis of colonic carcinoma, the feces of Western people apparently contain increased proportions of anaerobic bacteria and these anaerobes allegedly degrade cholate to deoxycholate which then may act as a cocarcinogen within the lumen of the colon. The addition of fiber to the diet presumably would decrease the prolonged transit time within the colon, inhibit this degradation of cholate, and also help to dilute an intraluminal "carcinogen." Other conceptual mechanisms attempt to explain the increased frequency of ischemic heart disease, hiatus hernia, appendicitis and inguinal hernia

largely on the basis of fiber-depleted diets in Western countries,
though it should be noted that no dietary allowance or dietary
requirement for fiber thus far has been established.

Most of these epidemiological studies have been reported in
the British literature, reflecting the influence of Burkitt's
observations. American physicians and scientists appear to have
directed little attention to these problems, and despite a considerable literature largely within the food industry, little
scientific and clinical attention has been directed to dietary
fiber and to the lack of fiber in the human diet. Yet fiber is a
food substance with many properties. It apparently is capable of
influencing intestinal and colonic function in many important ways.
What indeed is dietary fiber and what are its functions? How valid
are the epidemiological observations? Do they reflect an oversimplified view of the pathogenesis of complex illnesses undoubtedly
involving more than one mechanism? How can dietary fiber presumably
play a central role in the development of such diverse disorders as
cancer of the colon, hiatus hernia, ischemic heart disease and
diverticular disease of the large bowel? In the epidemiologic
comparison of many different population groups with varying economic, social, cultural and ethnic backgrounds, are there not other
as important if not more significant factors in the genesis of these
diseases?

To provide some answers to these challenging questions, a group
of scientific investigators, not all of whom were directly involved
in these fields of study, met for a one-day session on May 17, 1974.
The meeting was held in the Center for Continuing Education,
University of Chicago, under the sponsorship of the Gastroenterology
Section of the Department of Medicine at the University. To encourage free discussion, the meeting was limited to 34 participants
plus a small number of invited guests, representing the American
Medical Association, the Food and Drug Administration and companies
in the food industry. This volume represents a full record of the
invited papers and the discussions that followed their presentation.

The conference was oriented to dietary fiber and its possible
effects, especially upon colonic function and colonic disorders.
No attempt was made to extend the discussions to ischemic heart
disease or hiatus hernia. Thus, the program was divided into three
main sections, followed by a General Discussion and Summary:
I. Dietary fiber and interaction with bacteria and bile; II. Fiber
and colonic function; III. Fiber-deficient disorders of the colon.
The objectives of the meeting were: to define the limits of our
knowledge of fiber; to examine certain aspects of bowel function
in relation to the possible influences of dietary fiber; to challenge
the epidemiological observations mentioned earlier; to review the
evidence linking the lack of dietary fiber to certain colonic
disease and, most importantly, to encourage new studies of dietary

fiber and bowel disease. As was anticipated, the conference did
not provide decisive answers to these questions, although the
discussions amply confirmed the importance of the problem and its
broad scope.

Dr. Richard W. Reilly, Professor of Medicine at the University
of Chicago, planned and arranged the conference. To his organi-
zational skill a large share of the success of the meeting may be
attributed. Already a new cooperative group for the further study
of these problems in the United States is in the process of
organization. It seems safe to predict that there will be an
increased number of studies of dietary fiber and its relation to
health and disease in many important medical centers throughout
the world.

Contributing to these developments have been the enthusiastic
cooperation of all participants of the conference, and the efficient
help of Terese Denov, Conference Secretarial Coordinator, and all
the section secretaries who helped with the transcribing of manu-
scripts and the discussions. To all of these, we wish to express
our thanks and appreciation.

We are also greatly indebted to Franklin C. Bing, Ph.D., Vice-
President of Nutrition Dynamics, Inc., for helpful criticism and
editorial advice on the preparation of the volume.

Joseph B. Kirsner, M.D., Ph.D.

Louis Block Distinguished
Service Professor of Medicine
and Deputy Dean for Medical
Affairs, University of Chicago

Contents

PART I
DIETARY FIBER AND INTERACTION WITH BACTERIA AND BILE

DIETARY FIBER

D. M. Hegsted

Department of Nutrition, Harvard School of Public Health

Boston, Massachusetts

The Food and Drug Administration recently has published regulations on the type of nutritional material which may be listed on the labels of foods, and the mode of preparation, etc. A consideration of nutritional labeling emphasizes several important points with regard to dietary fiber.

In the first place, one danger of nutritional labeling is that it is primarily concerned with the essential nutrients--protein, carbohydrate, fat, vitamins and minerals. It is implied in this labeling that if the total intake of the various essential nutrients included on the label equals the recommended intake, then the nutritional needs are satisfied. This assumption is not true, since not all essential nutrients are noted on the label. The discussion of dietary fiber also emphasizes that consideration of essential nutrients alone is an inadequate evaluation of the diet.

The other point that nutritional labeling will emphasize is that if there is merit in dietary fiber, food manufacturers will wish to add fiber to food products. If so, they must be able to measure such fiber and to define its composition. If they desire to make health claims with regard to fiber, they also will have to state these claims clearly and with supporting evidence. The discussion today will indicate that we are not yet able to do so. We may agree, for example, that wheat bran is a good source of dietary fiber but many questions arise. Are all wheat brans the same? It seems obvious that they are not, but it will be necessary to state how they differ. Competition in the food industry will not allow the producers of wheat bran to preempt the field.

The major problem with the epidemiologic evidence is that the
changes in dietary practices which occur with industrial and
economic development tend to be similar in whatever geographical
area they occur. There is an increase in the consumption of
animal products, of fat, of sugar, of refined cereals, etc.
Figure 1 demonstrates data on fat and sugar consumption relative
to heart disease (McGandy, 1967). Obviously, when the changes in
consumption of two or more materials are highly correlated, the
data cannot prove whether either one or both are causally related
to the disease. Similar relationships usually can be shown for
non-food factors--changes in physical activity, increases in the
use of television, tin cans, automobiles, etc. Unless one can find
populations in which the individual factors to be studied are not
highly correlated, the epidemiologic evidence only suggests hypotheses which may then require investigation.

Many food tables provide data on crude fiber. Crude fiber is
defined empirically as organic material that survives hydrolysis
with dilute acid and alkali under specified conditions. It is a
crude estimate of the cellulose and lignin content. As will be
evident from the discussion today, there is no compelling reason
to think that this is what we are interested in when we are discussing dietary fiber.

Many food tables list total carbohydrate. This figure usually
is obtained by estimating differences, e.g., what is left after
water, protein, fat, ash, and crude fiber are subtracted, and
represents everything that has not already been accounted for.

The term "unavailable carbohydrate" also is inadequate, since
it includes not only the cellulose and lignin but a host of ill-
defined pentosans, galactosans, polyurans, etc. which are generally
grouped together as hemicellulose. In the past, at least, the
major reason for investigating the so-called "available" or
"unavailable" carbohydrate was to estimate the available energy in
the diet. Figure 2 is taken from Southgate (1969) and shows the
fractionation scheme he employed. Obviously, this approach is
empirical and while it does classify materials in foods there is
no particular reason to believe that materials grouped in these
categories have similar physiologic effects. We do not know
whether these different fractions have the same or different biologic activity, or whether materials within fractions have similar
or different activities.

The intestinal enzymes presumably can hydrolyze only the
simple sugars, dextrans and starch. These, then, are considered
to be "available" carbohydrates. However, a substantial proportion
of the so-called "unavailable" carbohydrate may disappear during
passage through the intestinal tract. We usually define digestion

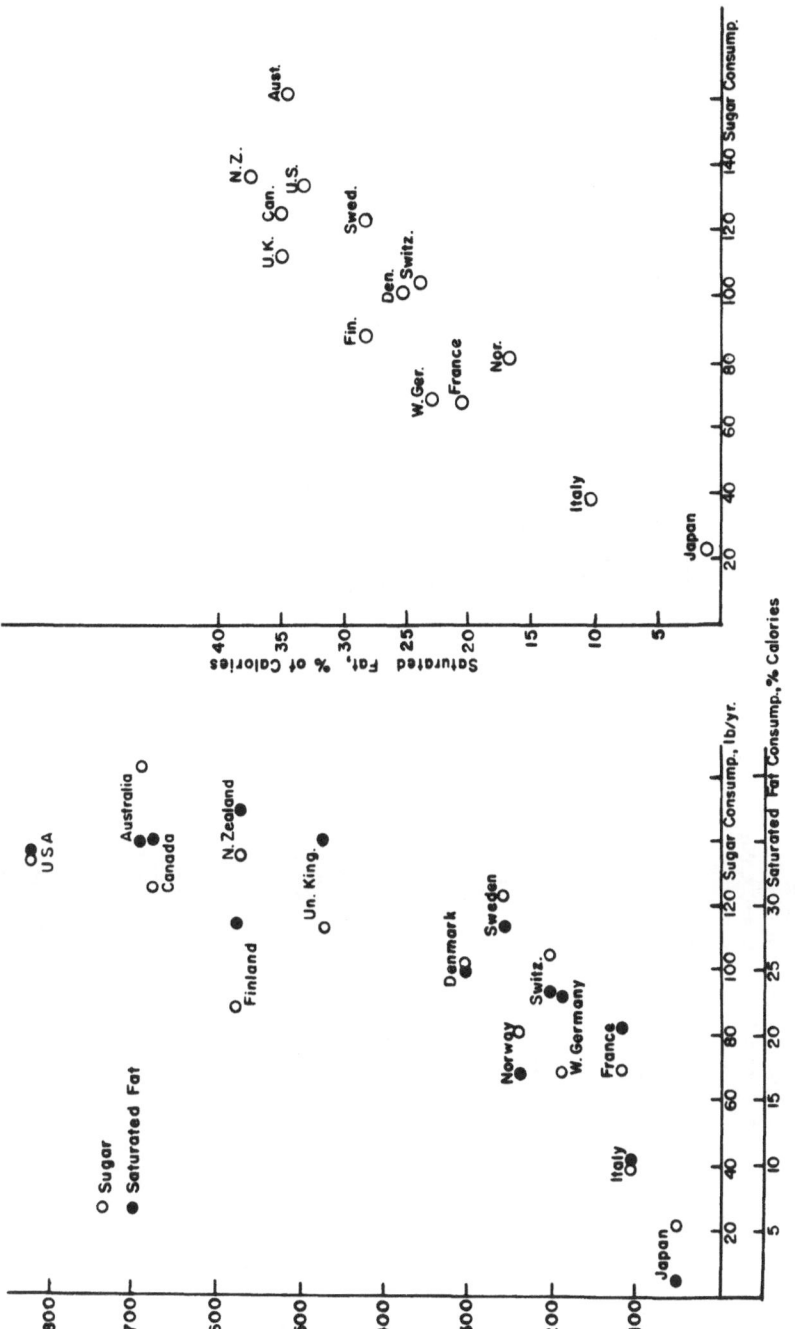

Fig. 1. Interrelations between sugar and saturated fat consumption and mortality from coronary heart disease (from McGandy, et al., 1967).

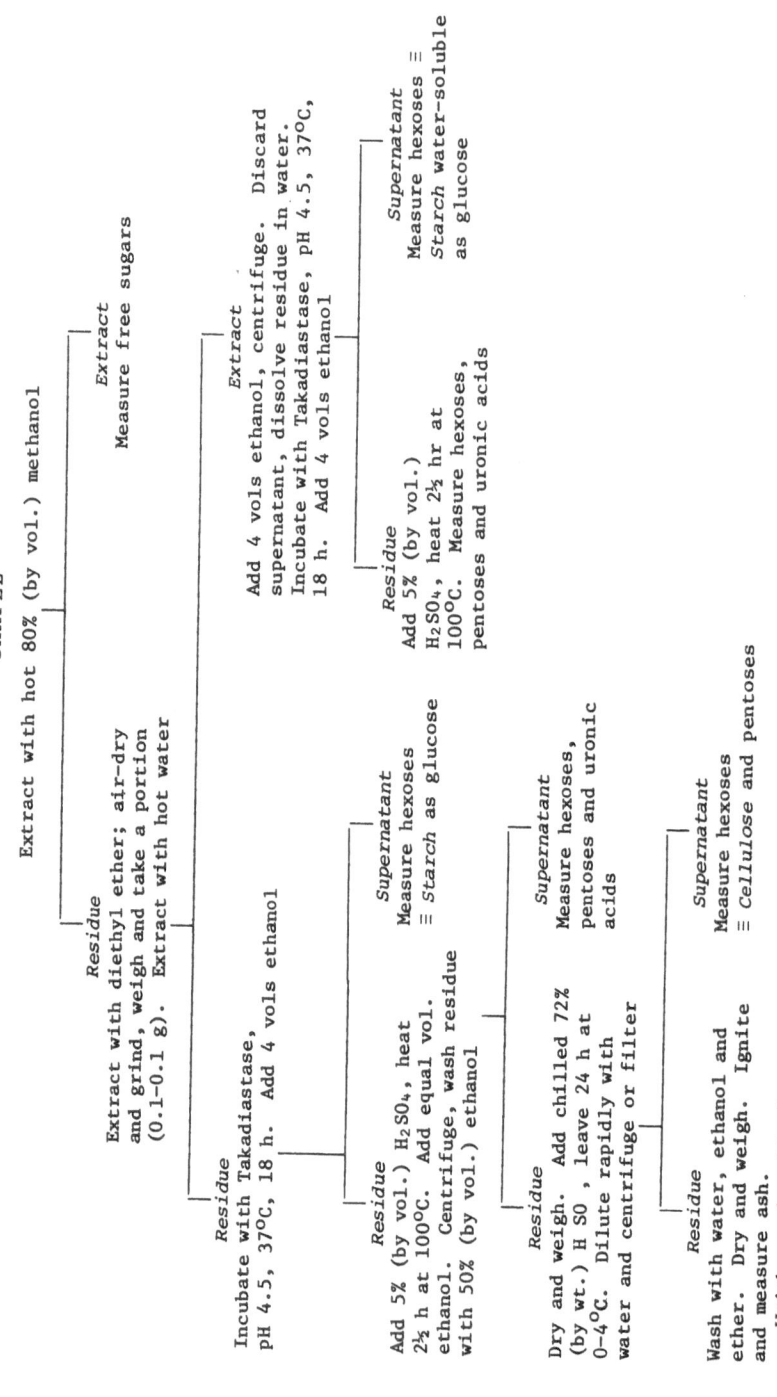

Fig. 2. Fractionation and analytical scheme for measuring unavailable carbohydrate and starch (from Southgate, 1969).

TABLE 1.   Intake and Fecal Excretion on Three Diets

	Diet 1		Diet 2		Diet 3	
	Intake	Excre-tion	Intake	Excre-tion	Intake	Excre-tion
Energy	2340	83	2490	127	2800	210
Protein as nitrogen	13.1	1.03	13.9	1.27	14.7	2.17
Fat	92	3.01	96.1	3.69	89.2	6.24
Pentosan	4.90	0.30	10.99	2.53	22.62	3.87
Cellulose	1.27	0.94	5.17	3.83	9.26	7.27

(from Southgate and Durnin, 1970)

as disappearance from the gastrointestinal tract, after ignoring
the fact that many compounds are secreted into the gut and reabsorbed to varying degrees, that much of the fecal material is of
bacterial origin, etc.

Some of the results published by Southgate and Durnin (1970)
are shown in Table 1. They investigated the effects of three
different diets, one low in fiber, another with substantial amounts
of fruits and vegetables, and another with still more dietary fiber.
Note that by using these analytical procedures a substantial amount

TABLE 2.   Digestibility of Three Diets

	Diet 1	Diet 2	Diet 3
Energy	96.5 (95.5 – 97.3)	94.9 (93.8 – 96.4)	92.5 (91.5 – 93.2)
Protein	92.1 (87.1 – 95.7)	90.8 (87.0 – 95.0)	85.2 (82.7 – 87.6)
Fat	96.7 (95.7 – 97.6)	96.2 (94.9 – 97.0)	93.0 (91.7 – 94.3)
Pentosan	93.9 (91.7 – 96.1)	77.0 (72.9 – 83.7)	92.9 (80.5 – 84.0)
Cellulose	25.5 (2.2 – 48.4)	26.0 (6.6 – 40.1)	21.5 (10.8 – 31.9)

(from Southgate and Durnin, 1970)

of the so-called unavailable carbohydrate disappears, including a
significant amount of the cellulose.

Table 2 shows the calculated digestibility of the various
fractions. Note that the total energy that was digested or disappeared fell slightly as the fiber content of the diets increased.
On the basis of this observation, Southgate and others have concluded that the "unavailable" carbohydrate does not contribute to
the energy supply. One should also note, however, that the digestibility of the fat and protein fell. The increase in the fecal
content of these materials accounts for approximately half of the
increase in the energy content of the feces. The source of the
fat and the protein, however, i.e., whether they represent the fat
and the protein in the fiber source or an effect of the fiber on
general fat and protein digestion, is unknown. Thus, the data
indicate no net increase in available energy when these "unavailable"
carbohydrate sources are included in the diet, but a substantial
amount disappears and apparently is metabolized. Presumably much
of this "digestion" is accomplished by bacterial action with the
formation of short-chain fatty acids which then are metabolized.

Figure 3 indicates the composition of a variety of sources of
dietary fiber which were fed by Williams and Olmsted (1936).
Figure 4 indicates the amount of so-called "indigestible residue"
which was fed, the changes in stool weight, and the amount of the

MATERIALS ADDED TO THE BASAL DIET	WHEAT BRAN	ALFALFA LEAF MEAL	CARROTS	CORN GERM MEAL	COTTON SEED HULL	SUGAR BEET PULP	CANNED PEAS	CABBAGE	AGAR AGAR	CELLU FLOUR
	Per cent	Per cent	Per cent	Per cent	Per cent	Per cent	Per cent	Per cent	Per cent	Per cent
Cellulose	16.9	32.5	23.2	15.8	19.4	34.2	35.0	29.5	0.0	78.8
Lignin	7.8	15.0	3.4	2.4	20.8	2.5	1.7	2.6	0.0	0.0
Hemicellulose (S)	35.2	15.5	20.7	28.9	30.9	20.4	8.8	19.8	81.0	16.9
Hemicellulose (L)	0.0	3.7	8.1	1.9	0.6	8.8	2.1	8.5	....	0.0
Starch	6.6	2.5	0.7	10.9	3.2	1.8	13.6	0.0	0.0	0.0
Protein (N×6.25)	12.3	12.4	7.8	18.6	7.3	8.5	16.5	10.8	1.6	0.0
Moisture (110°)	8.9	6.5	11.1	7.5	8.2	7.9	7.5	10.0	13.5	3.0
Ash (red heat)	4.4	2.3	5.8	5.5	1.8	2.3	2.2	3.8	3.4	0.1
Soluble in alcohol-benzene	3.5	9.0	15.2	7.2	7.0	9.8	9.7	12.5	0.0	0.0
Total	95.6	99.4	96.0	98.7	99.2	96.2	97.1	97.5	99.5	98.8

(L) Soluble in solutions pH 8.
(S) Insoluble in solutions pH 8.

Fig. 3. Composition of various sources of dietary fiber. (from
Williams and Olmsted, 1936).

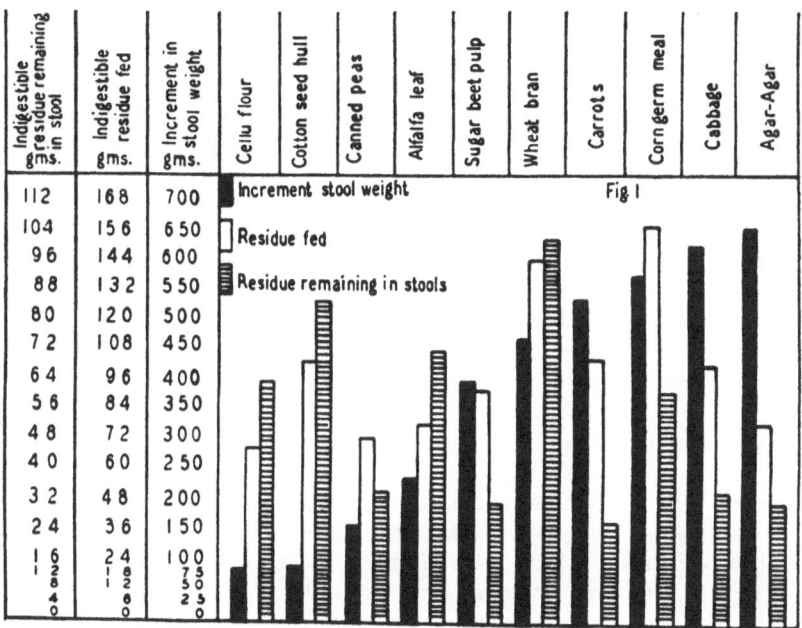

Fig. 4. Changes in stool weight and residue remaining in stools compared to the amount of residue fed (from Williams & Olmsted, 1936).

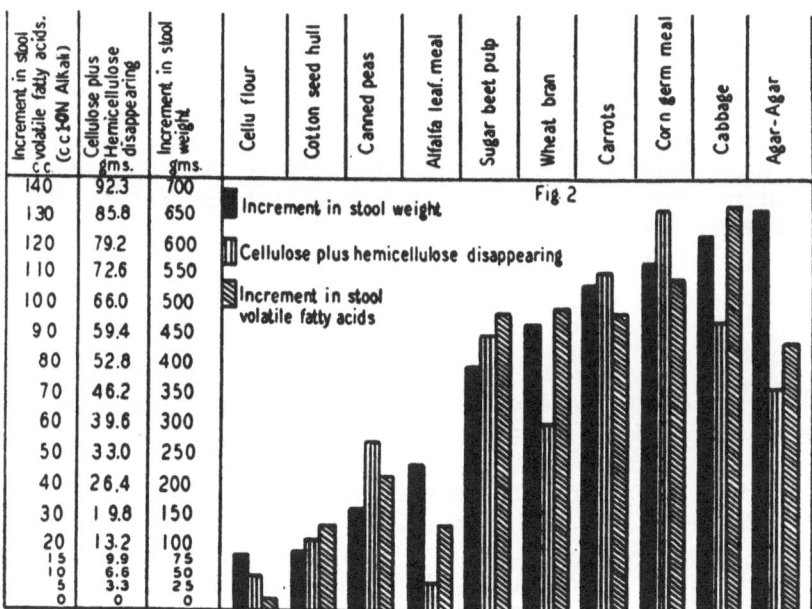

Fig. 5. Stool weight in relation to cellulose and hemicellulose which disappeared and fecal short-chain fatty acids (from Williams & Olmsted, 1936).

residue remaining in the stools. The materials are arranged in order of the increment in stool weight. There appears to be little relationship between these values. Note, for example, that nearly all of the residue fed as wheat bran was recoverable in the stools, yet carrots produced equally large stools even though less residue was fed and most of it disappeared.

Figure 5 shows data from the same experiment. There appears to be some relationship between the amount of hemicellulose and cellulose which disappeared and the stool weight. Furthermore, there may be some relationship between the stool content of volatile fatty acids and the stool weight. This would suggest that it is not the amount of indigestible residue which remains in the stool that determines volume, but rather the metabolic products of the digestion of some of these materials.

The conclusions to be reached from such observations are that dietary fiber is as yet undefined and non-measurable. We do not know whether we are dealing with materials that have a variety of physiologic actions or a variety of materials which have similar actions. We do not know whether the effects of dietary fiber are directly attributable to the fiber or to the materials derived from fiber.

In this field we appear to be at a stage in our research comparable to that existing in the 1930's when the only vitamin B available was a crude material that subsequently was shown to consist of a variety of components with differing physiologic effects. Progress in the field of dietary fiber probably will depend upon improved analytical methods, upon the development of biologic test systems to quantitate the effects, and upon the separation and the testing of various fractions in what now is called "dietary fiber."

REFERENCES

McGandy, R. B., Hegsted, D. M., and Stare, F. J., 1967, Dietary fats, carbohydrates and atherosclerotic vascular disease, New Engl. J. Med., 277:417, 469.

Southgate, D. A. T., 1969, Determination of carbohydrates in foods, II. Unavailable carbohydrates, J. Sci., Food Agri., 20:331-335.

Southgate, D. A. T., and Durnin, J. V. G. A., 1970, Caloric conversion factors. An experimental reassessment of the factors used in the calculation of the energy value of human diets, Brit. J. Nutr., 24:517-535.

Williams, R. D. and Olmsted, W. H., 1936, the effect of cellulose,
    hemicellulose and lignin on the weight of the stool: A
    contribution to the study of laxation in man, J. Nutr.,
    11:433-449.

DISCUSSION

A. F. Hofmann: Dr. Hegsted began with a chemical definition
of fiber that was operational, being based on solubility. There
obviously is an enormous amount of work to be done on the chemical
characterization of fiber. Apparently such has not been done.
Is that correct?

D. M. Hegsted: As far as I can tell, it has not been done.
Unfortunately, it seems to me that in some ways, it is almost an
impossible job unless we can develop appropriate biological test
systems. An attempt could be made to characterize all the carbohydrates and other compounds in a crude material, but this is
not the best approach. I can remember somebody stating 30 years
ago "if you want to know what nutrients animals need, all you
have to do is to take corn and identify everything in it and you
will then know what all the requirements are." That approach would
not have worked. We need a test system that will do more than
simply identify everything that we might consider to be fiber.

A. H. Hofmann: There are at least two aspects to this problem.
One is to define what we do not know and the other is to select
research priorities according to what is possible. Chemical technics for determining the primary structure of polymers are evolving
and are becoming automated. No one would have imagined 20 years
ago that we would be sequencing proteins. We soon could have
automated technics for defining the chemical structures of the
individual constituents of bran. Would it be your opinion that
this is a worthy goal when carried out in conjunction with appropriate bioassays?

D. M. Hegsted: I think that the technics probably are
available if somebody would put as much effort into this area as
is directed to protein synthesis.

A. I. Mendeloff: I should like to read into the record a
letter in Lancet of March 23, 1974, by Dr. Hugh Trowell, which
comments on dietary fiber (DF): "In view of discussions held with
some biochemists and nutritionists in the United States, DF appears
to contain the following groups of substances." I will not read
his letter in detail; he lists six groups of substances which are
agreed upon apparently as a result of recent data which I have not
seen published. Trowell defines DF as "1) structural poly-

saccharides; 2) lignins; 3) unavailable lipids including waxes and cutins; 4) probably unavailable nitrogen associated with fiber; 5) trace elements associated with fiber; and 6) probably-unidentified enzymes, minerals, salts, and other substances present largely in a relatively unavailable form in the vegetable cell wall. The role of phytic acid and calcium awaits full evaluation by long-term studies in man." He then points out that if standard foods are analyzed by conventional technics, the values that emerge are far lower than those identified by his system.

A. F. Hofmann: This is an heterogenous operational definition. We also need a chemical definition, especially for the polysaccharide component.

G. J. Devroede: This is a crucial question for clinical studies. We have written to a random sample of dietetic departments in Canadian hospitals to learn how they define a "low residue diet." (Figure 1) There are tremendous differences from hospital

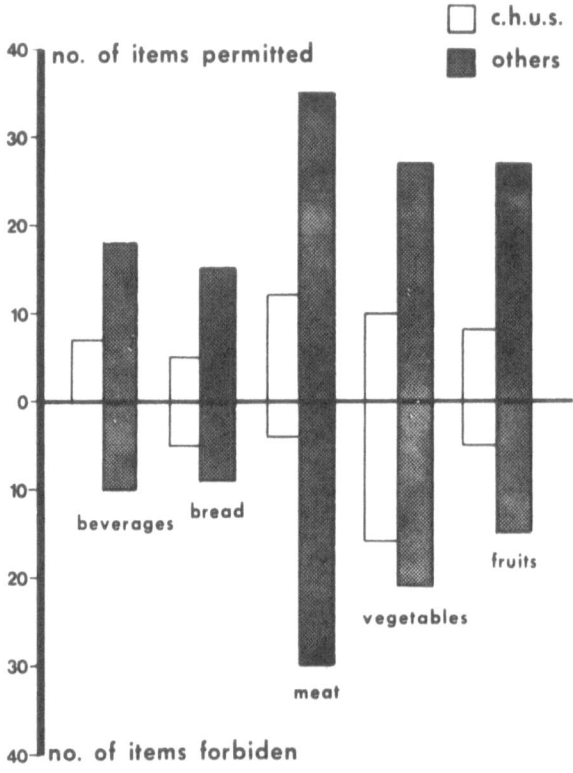

Fig. 1. The low-residue dietary items forbidden in University Hospital (C.H.U.S.) compared to other Canadian hospitals.

to hospital. We will talk about clinical trials with dietary fiber later and it is important that we keep these great differences in definition in mind.

A. F. Hofmann: I would like to ask Dr. Levitt to discuss how we might assess digestibility of fiber. Let us assume, for the moment, that the fiber is carbohydrate.

M. D. Levitt: I gather that Dr. Hofmann is referring to our use of breath tests in the study of the absorption of carbohydrates. One technic would be to develop a ^{14}C labeled fiber and feed it to individuals. The quantity of $^{14}CO_2$ excreted on the breath would then be an indication of whether the fibers could be digested and then metabolized by either the body or the intestinal bacteria. My own studies with hydrogen gas also would suggest that measurement of the rate at which hydrogen is excreted by the lungs provides a useful indicator of bacterial fermentation of carbohydrate. Since human cellular metabolism does not make hydrogen gas, the rate of hydrogen excretion after fiber ingestion might provide an indication of the ability of the bacteria to digest fiber.

A. F. Hofmann: Dr. Hegsted, are there not several biological stations that raise plants completely labeled with ^{14}C? Could fiber from such plants be made available to clinical investigators to test this point?

D. M. Hegsted: If you know what you are interested in, and can isolate it, then you could measure its metabolism and digestibility. Of course, it is only a suppostion that digestibility is really what we are interested in. The digestion products of the indigestible material also may have important effects. However, if appropriately labeled materials were available, they certainly would be helpful in metabolic studies.

B. H. Ershoff: I should like to expand on Dr. Hegsted's remark about different kinds of fibers having different kinds of effects. The analogy to the B vitamins is a good one. There is at least one major difference, however, between the function of plant fibers and that of B vitamins. The latter are essential components of the intracellular metabolism of each cell of the body; the plant fibers, on the other hand, exert their effects outside of the tissue cell and to a large extent, if not entirely, within the intestinal tract per se.

There is good evidence that dietary fiber can promote health by at least three different mechanisms: First, in regulating normal bowel function, and this is largely the topic of the conference today. In this category, we include such effects as the bulk-forming capacity of plant fibers and the resulting increase

in stool weight, promotion of regularity, rapid transit time, etc.
A second mechanism relates to the hypocholesterolemic and anti-
atherosclerotic effects of certain dietary fibers. The literature
in this field recently has been reviewed by Trowell (1972). A third
mechanism is by the antitoxic effect of plant fibers.

During the past 20 years a considerable volume of data has
been published (Ershoff, in press) indicating that a number of
drugs, chemicals, and food additives which are without deleterious
effect, or have very little deleterious effect when fed at certain
doses to animals on a high-fiber diet, can cause marked toxic
effects such as growth retardation, tissue pathology, and even
death when fed at the same dose levels to animals on a low-fiber
diet.

There is evidence that plant fibers with antitoxic activity
may be without hypocholesterolemic activity and that the converse
also may be true. Thus methoxy pectin (i.e., pectin with a
methoxyl content of 5.0% or less) had marked activity in counteracting the growth-retardation and other toxic effects in rats fed
a purified low-fiber diet containing 5% sodium cyclamate, but was
without activity in counteracting the increment in plasma and liver
cholesterol, and liver total lipids induced by cholesterol feeding
in the rat. Similarly, sodium alginate had marked activity in
counteracting the growth retardation and other toxic effects in
rats fed a purified, low-fiber diet containing 15% of the non-ionic
surface-active agent Tween 60 but was without activity in counteracting the increment in plasma and liver cholesterol and liver
total lipids induced by cholesterol feeding in the rat. Conversely,
locust bean gum which had marked activity as a hypocholesterolemic
agent in the rat was virtually devoid of activity in counteracting
the toxic effects induced by sodium cyclamate when incorporated at
a 5% level in a purified, low-fiber diet in the rat.

Now, of course, the question arises as to whether the effects
of various plant fiber-containing materials are due to the plant
fibers per se or to accessory substances that may be present in
them. Here the chemist comes to our aid. Sodium carboxymethylcellulose is an artificial gum widely used in the food industry,
which is produced by the introduction of a controlled number of
sodium carboxymethyl groups into the cellulose molecule. When
cellulose reacts to form carboxymethylcellulose, water solubility
and other desirable physical properties are acquired which are
dependent on the degree of substitution, the uniformity of distribution of the substituent carboxymethyl groups on the polymer
chain, the degree of polymerization, and physical characteristics
such as particle size, shape and density. These preparations contain virtually no trace elements, vitamins, or other nutrients;
their chemical nature is clearly defined; and it is possible to

duplicate with some of these chemically-produced gums the physiological effects obtained with a number of natural gums and fibers.

These findings appear to indicate that the physiologic effects
of various dietary fibers are due at least in part to the chemical
and physical properties of their fibers (including such properties
as swelling power, ion-exchange capacity, etc.). Inasmuch as the
antitoxic efficacy of plant fibers can be evaluated in rats and
mice in two weeks or less and their hypocholesterolemic activity
in four weeks or less, these procedures would appear to be of
value as bioassays for evaluating the physiologic properties and
therapeutic potential of various plant fibers.

REFERENCES

Trowell, H., 1972, Ischemic heart disease and dietary fiber, Am.
    J. Clin. Nutr., 25:926-932.

Ershoff, B. H., Antitoxic effects of plant fiber, Am. J. Clin.
    Nutr., in press.

THE INTERRELATIONSHIP BETWEEN BILE ACIDS, BACTERIA AND DIETARY FIBER

M. A. Eastwood

Wolfson Gastrointestinal Laboratory, Western General Hospital

Edinburgh, Scotland

We have approached this problem as one of physical chemistry and have tried to define the physical characteristics of dietary fiber rather than concentrate on the chemical identification of its constituents (Eastwood, 1973). Current thinking suggests that most of the biological activity of dietary fiber occurs in the colon. It is possible to depict such events as a triangle, in which there is an interaction between bacteria, bile and fiber, all complicated by time spent in the colon (Figure 1).

INFLUENCE OF TIME

First, I would like to discuss the effect of intestinal transit time upon fecal bacteria and bile acids, the transit time being the time taken for barium-impregnated plastic markers to pass from the mouth to the anus (Hunter, et al., 1969).

Two groups of normal individuals were compared, one group in which the transit time was less than 24 hours, the other with a transit time of more than 50 hours. The fecal bacterial flora was essentially the same quantitatively and qualitatively. Similarly, the mean stool weight, dry weight of stool, total fecal bile acid output, and the deoxycholic and lithocholic acid content of the feces were not significantly different in the two groups.

INTERPLAY BETWEEN BACTERIA AND FIBER

Dietary plant fiber will vary from plant to plant; with the age, type, and variety of plant, and also with the anatomical source of the tissue. Rapidly growing plant tissues contain substantial amounts of pectins and hemicelluloses; the more mature plant tissues will be predominantly lignin and cellulose. Very few data are available on the interplay between bacteria and fiber for human nutrition. It is possible that polysaccharides are subject to bacterial degradation in the colon (Cumming, 1973) but lignins are not modified by bacteria. It is not known how bacteria align themselves on the fibers--whether they are adsorbed to the fiber or are randomly distributed throughout the heterogeneous phases. Many bacteria produce extracellular enzymes that will permeate into the system so that there will be remote as well as intracellular metabolism.

INTERPLAY BETWEEN BACTERIA AND BILE ACIDS

There are two modifications to bile acid conjugates which are important: one of these is a robust reaction, deconjugation with removal of the glycine and taurine conjugate; the other is a 7alpha-dehydroxylation (Norman & Shorb, 1962) that is sensitive to a variety of inhibitory situations which may include rapid transit through the colon and high concentrations of bile acids (Kern, 1973). At the concentration of bile acids normally found in the stool (2-5 mM) there is an initial stage when deconjugation takes place which is followed by 7alpha-dehydroxylation, without killing the bacteria; deconjugation, however, is unaffected (Mitchell, et al., 1974).

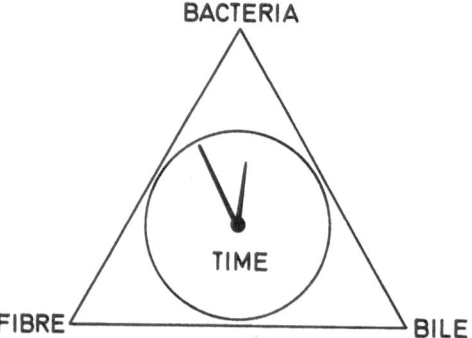

Fig. 1. Dietary fiber, bile and bacteria interrelated and these interrelationships affected by time.

INTERPLAY BETWEEN BILE ACIDS AND FIBER

Bile acids are adsorbed onto dietary fibers so that the bile acid conjugates that are found in the duodenum are the least strongly adsorbed. The secondary bile acids generated in the colon by bacterial activity are the most strongly adsorbed. This adsorption is pH-dependent and seems to be associated with suppression of ionization within the dietary fiber (Eastwood & Hamilton, 1968).

The importance of phases may be illustrated by the diarrhea associated with ileal resection. In this condition, there is a high concentration of bile acids capable of inhibiting 7alpha-dehydroxylation. The stools from these patients contain chenodeoxycholic and cholic acid. In some patients, successful treatment with cholestyramine or lignin coincides with the appearance of secondary bile acids with no change in the total amount of bile acids excreted in the stool. In diverticular disease, there is a small stool with a high concentration of bile acids approaching 10 mM, which in vitro is capable of inhibiting 7alpha-dehydroxylation, yet in this situation there is no such inhibition.

The pool size of bile acids in the small intestine of a fiber-free diet is approximately 7 mg with a ratio of cholic acid to dihydroxy acids of 2.5:1. If cellulose or wheat bran is added to the diet, then the pool of bile acids in the small intestine increases (Boyd & Eastwood, 1968).

Conjugated bile acids in the jejunum are involved in micelle formation and fat absorption. An unknown proportion of bile acid conjugates are absorbed in the ileum, and the remainder will pass into the cecum, associated in part with the dietary fiber. Within the cecum there is the generation of less-soluble bile acids which are more readily adsorbed to fiber. While some of these bile acids will be reabsorbed and pass to the liver via the portal vein, the remainder will be excreted in the feces. Thus a potential exists for altering the amount of bile acids passing out in the feces by using the appropriate fiber. In man, there is a linear relationship between the daily total fecal bile acid excretion and the wet-weight of feces of normal individuals eating their habitual diets (Eastwood, et al., 1973). It is possible that by increasing the stool weight, perhaps by manipulation of the dietary fiber intake both qualitatively and quantitatively, fecal bile acid output might similarly increase.

PHYSICAL CHARACTERISTICS OF FIBER

Wettability. This is the capacity of the fiber to absorb

water when exposed to excess water. Hydrophilic substances like
hemi-cellulose and pectin will accumulate water, whereas lignin,
which is relatively hydrophobic, will not. In considering dietary
sources of fiber, the amount of fiber taken with a raw vegetable
will vary; turnip and celery contain 4-6% dry material whereas bran
contains 85% dry material. The capacity of dietary fiber to adsorb
water varies with the type of fiber. We have studied this capacity
in fiber obtained from plants that have been frozen to disrupt the
cells, washed with water (30-40°C) to remove water-soluble materials,
and then dried with acetone. This fiber, free of protein, fat and
water-soluble carbohydrates resembles the fiber passing from the
ileum into the cecum. Such fiber from wheat bran holds five times
its own weight of water, yet fiber from carrot or turnip will hold
between 27-30 times its own weight in water. Thus, if allowance
is made for the fiber content of the original raw plant and the
water-holding capacity of the dried material, 100 g of bran, despite
its modest water-holding capacity, will have a superior overall
hydrophilic property (450 g water per fiber in 100 g raw material).
Mango (320 g water); carrot (220 g water); apple (180 g water) and
brussel sprouts (170 g water) have potent hydrophilic properties
that can be utilized in increasing stool weight (MConnell, et al.,
1974).

Cation Exchange Capacity. Fiber, and presumably the polysaccharide component, has cation exchange capacity of 2.5 meq/g dry
fiber, approximately the same as commercially-available weak cation
exchangers (McConnell, et al., 1974).

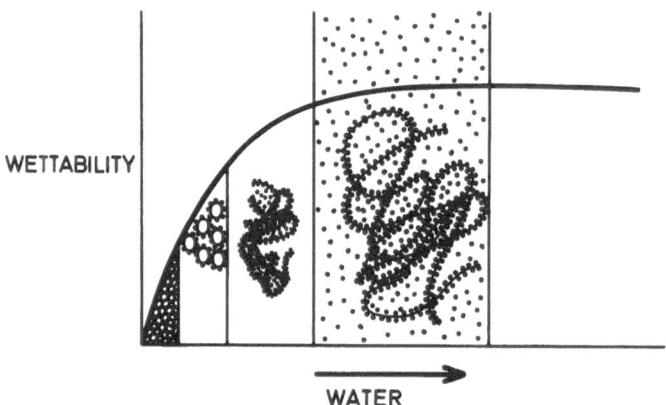

WETTABILITY

WATER

Fig. 2. Stages in wetting of fiber from anhydrous (section 1);
surface water (section 2); interstitial water (section 3); free
water co-inciding with saturation of the fiber with water
(section 4).

FECES A HETEROGENEOUS SYSTEM

Feces consist of a matrix of fiber hydrated with water. The water is adsorbed to the fiber surface, entrapped in the interstices of the fiber and, in a diarrheal stool, also exists as free water (Figure 2). Other constituents of the stool will be adsorbed to the fiber or distributed through the stool according to size, configuration, solubility, electrostatic charge and other physical characteristics. That is, there will be biological sieving.

Evidence that feces are not homogeneous in phases is given by experiments with water-soluble (polyethylene glycol 4000) and water-insoluble (chromium sesquioxide) intestinal markers (Findlay, et al., 1974). It is possible to mark the stool contents simultaneously with these two markers; the PEG 4000 will mark most of the liquid phase (limited by molecular weight and intrusion into the fiber interstices) and the Cr_2O_3 will mark the solid phase. If there is true mixing between the two phases during the first 5-7 days of administration, then the PEG 4000 and Cr_2O_3 will appear in the stool together (Figure 3). If, however, there is streaming, then one phase will come through at a different rate from the other. In normal individuals, there is a linear relationship between Cr_2O_3 and PEG 4000 marking with a slope that is virtually unity (Findlay, et al., 1974). If one feeds these normal individuals wheat bran, there is stratification of the feces after one month, so that Cr_2O_3 is excreted much faster than PEG 4000. The converse applies to individuals with diverticular disease. In

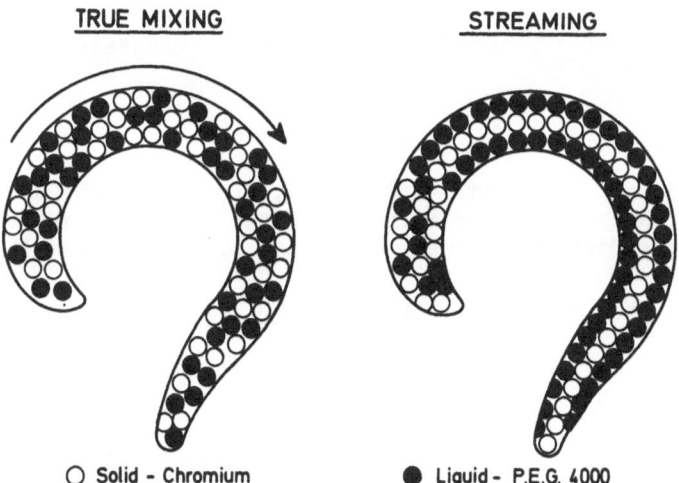

TRUE MIXING   STREAMING

○ Solid - Chromium   ● Liquid - P.E.G. 4000

Fig. 3. Phenomena of true mixing and streaming of solid phase (with Cr_2O_3) and liquid phase (PEG 4000) in the colon.

their untreated state they excrete Cr_2O_3 faster than PEG 4000, but when wheat bran is given with resulting symptomatic relief and return of the colonic manometric pressures to normal, then the slope of the graph of excreted Cr_2O_3 to PEG 4000 moves towards unity (Findlay, et al., 1974).

What is probably happening in normal individuals is that the Cr_2O_3 is associated with the surface of the fiber while the PEG 4000 equates with most of the water phase, and both phases move together through the colon. In diverticular disease, there is increased colonic pressure and expression of the aqueous phase both backwards and forwards, so that there is some delay in PEG excretion.

In summary, the interrelationships between fiber, bacteria and bile are complex. Fiber has physical characteristics of wettability, cation exchange and bile acid adsorption. Bacteria metabolize both fiber and bile, and bile influences bacterial metabolism. We can only guess at the influence of surfaces, spaces, water distribution, time, concentration, redox potential and pH in such a complex.

I would agree entirely with Dr. Hegsted about the embryonic stage of our knowledge of fiber. Our enlightenment about vitamins was the result of work by biochemists, and I suspect that the fiber story will rely heavily upon physical chemists for its clarification.

I am grateful to Drs. Falkehag, Findlay, Mitchell, McRae and McConnell for their guidance and contributions. This work is supported in part by the British Nutrition Foundation.

REFERENCES

Boyd, G. S. and Eastwood, M. A., 1968, Studies on the quantitative distribution of bile salts along the rat small intestine under varying dietary regimes, Biochiem. Biophys. Acta, 152:159-164.

Cumming, J. H., 1973, Dietary fiber, Gut, 14:69-81.

Eastwood, M. A., 1973, Vegetable fiber; its physical properties, Proc. Nutr. Soc., 22:137-143.

Eastwood, M. A. and Hamilton, D., 1968, Studies on the adsorption of bile salts to non-absorbed components of diet, Biochiem. Biophys. Acta, 152:165-173.

Eastwood, M. A., Kirkpatrick, J. R., Mitchell, W. D., Bone, A. and
    Hamilton, T., 1973, Effects of dietary supplements of wheat
    bran in feces and bowel function, Brit. Med. J., 4:392-394.

Findlay, J. M., Smith, A. N., Mitchell, W. D., Anderson, A. J. and
    Eastwood, M. A., 1974, Effects of unprocessed bran on colon
    function in normal subjects and in diverticular disease,
    Lancet, i:146-149.

Hunter, J. M., Leonard-Jones, J. E., Young, A. C., 1969, A new
    method for studying gut transit times using radio-opaque
    markers, Gut, 10:842-847.

Kern, F. Jr., 1973, Disappearance of deoxycholic acid after ileal
    resection, Gastroenterology, 64:123-127.

McConnell, A. A., Eastwood, M. A. and Mitchell, W. D., 1974, Phy-
    sical characteristics of vegetable foodstuffs that could
    influence bowel function, J. Sci. Food and Agric. (in the
    press).

Mitchell, W. D., Findlay, J. M., MacRae, R., Eastwood, M. A. and
    Anderson, R., 1974, in the press.

Norman, A. and Shorb, M. S., 1962, In vitro formation of deoxy-
    cholic and lithocholic acid by human intestinal micro-
    organisms, Proc. Soc. Exp. Biol., 110:552-555.

DISCUSSION

M. H. Floch: I would like to have your opinion of our ability
to truly assess the bacterial variations and their significance.
In my opinion, after years of study, our technics are still not
critical enough to indicate whether the bacterial content is or is
not significant on a quantitative basis.

M. A. Eastwood: I agree entirely. One is limited in the
classification of these bacteria by methodology that was developed
for quite different purposes. In looking for functional differences
within these groups, we are not entirely certain what questions to
ask.

A. F. Hofmann: Dr. Eastwood, it seems to me that what is
needed are the binding adsorption isotherms of the different bile
acids in small intestinal content as it changes in composition from
the duodenum to the rectum. Is not that the information we need
initially?

M. A. Eastwood: This is very difficult information to
secure for a number of reasons. The characteristics of the intestinal contents along the gut will change. The physical charcter-
istics of the fiber will be dictated by digestion of the fiber and
other smaller molecules and by the osmolality of the fluid of the
intestinal tract, and it will be modified by competing adsorption
of other materials to the fiber. Adsorption also will be affected
by bacterial metabolism of the fiber. When all of these factors
are added together there are too many variables. Much in vitro
work still remains to be completed.

I. H. Rosenberg: It will be important to learn not only the
capacity of fiber, in its various forms down the intestinal tract,
for bile salt binding but also the equilibrium characteristics.
In addition, we should know the extent to which bacterial effects
still occur as well as the extent to which osmotic and other
physiologic effects of bile salts on the gut can still occur.

M. A. Eastwood: I agree. This is clearly proved by newly-
developed lignin derivatives which demonstrate good binding capa-
cities in in vitro experiments but which have proved disappointing
in animal experiments. The binding by lignin is a hydrophobic
adsorption and hence is different and less strong than the electrostatic adsorption by cholestyramine. The physical chemistry of
this adsorption is, however, complicated.

M. M. Schuster: In the streaming effect that was sbserved in
diverticular disease, what was the differential passage of solids
and liquids? Was transit time altered more greatly for solids
than for liquids and, specifically, was this localized in different
areas of the colon? We know that there is a differential in
motility between the proximal and distal colon.

M. A. Eastwood: It is difficult to cite an exact figure
because these figures are accumulations. There seems to be a 30%
difference in transit time between these two phases. We obviously
cannot measure at various points along the intestinal tract, but
we know that the prime holdup in diverticular disease is in the
descending colon, so that it is with distal circular muscle spasm
that these streaming effects become apparent.

A. F. Hofmann: May I comment on something that I think is
important? In talking about bile acid concentrations in the stool,
we must be very clear about the equation denominator. Individuals
in the United States normally excrete 100-200 g of stool and we
eliminate approximately 1 mM of bile acids per day. The concentration of bile acids, if they were all in solution, would approxi-
mate 10 mM, which is not really different from that of patients
with bile acid diarrhea. Yet the physical state is totally

different. We must specify the physical state of bile acids. This
single term of concentration is very misleading. For example, the
claim that bile acids are present in lower concentration in the
feces of Africans who eat high residue diets can be predicted,
since the denominator is larger.

M. A. Eastwood: I agree entirely, but I do not know quite
how to describe concentration in feces, and yet we cannot speak of
a gradient of concentration along phases, fiber, organic material,
bacteria and water. The amount of bile acid per unit of stool is
greater in diverticular disease than in an equivalent normal stool.
The watery stool of ileal resection has a considerable content of
bile acid per g of stool. In the ileal resection stool most of
the bile acids are associated with the solid phase. How this
solid phase influences the fecal contents in diverticular disease,
in ileal resection, or in normal subjects, is not yet clear. If
bile acids are concentrated in the fiber or bacterial phase, then
to discuss concentration is misleading. Similarly, the aqueous
phase will vary in its nature-adsorbed, interstitial and free,
each phase perhaps exerting a different influence on stool characteristics.

M. M. Stanley: Your remark that concentration is only one
part of the answer to the problem also applies to bacteria. Were
your figures on bacteria for concentration alone, or were they
corrected for stool weight? This would make considerable difference
and the same factors might also apply to bacteria and bile acids.

M. A. Eastwood: No, these figures represent concentrations.
We have not corrected for the stool weight.

M. M. Stanley: Would it make any difference to your conclusions if these figures were expressed as numbers of organisms
excreted per day?

M. A. Eastwood: No, it would not. We have made such calcu-
lations for normal subjects and patients with diverticular disease
and they seem to excrete the same amount per day.

S. L. Gorbach: Having listened to the problems of defining
fiber, I have the same feeling of frustration about defining the
normal intestinal flora. Metchnikoff started the controversy by
suggesting that changes in the flora prolonged life, and ever
since then every benefit and malady that seems to occur to man
has been ascribed to changes in flora.

It is, however, very difficult to quantitate the bacterial
flora. I noted that some of your counts of obligate anaerobes,
for example, were lower than those given in other reports. It may

be in this area that your data differ from other observations made
in the past. For example, our group and others have noted that in
patients with severe diarrhea, such as cholera, or E. coli infection,
or diarrhea induced by perfusion of saline into the bowel, there is
a marked decrease in total cultivable anaerobes. This finding has
been confirmed in the United States where lesser degrees of diarrhea
also have been associated with a reduction in the number of anaerobic organisms that are recoverable in the feces. Now this is a
rather important area because anaerobic organisms are extremely
metabolic; they are proteolytic; and they are capable of performing
several of the alterations of the bile acid ring as well as deconjugation.

It may be that in your patients with ileal resection, lignin
is reducing the transit through the colon. This situation may
allow more organisms to grow, organisms that are difficult to
quantitate; or it may allow organisms to metabolize in a way that
they would not do if the colonic contents were moving more rapidly.
There is some information to suggest that Eh (the oxidation-
reduction potential) of the bowel is elevated in acute diarrhea.
Normally the Eh of the colon is approximately -250 mv and in
diarrhea it may be -75 mv. This change would alter the metabolic
activity of obligate anaerobes.

The other interesting point is that diet may affect not only
the quantitative aspects of the flora but also the qualitative
ability to metabolize bile salts and steroids. I do not know what
effects lignin would have on the metabolic properties of the flora.
I would point out that the metabolic potential of bacteria can
change by providing the micro-organisms with substrate due to
enzyme adaption.

BILE SALTS AND FIBER

K. W. Heaton

Bristol Royal Infirmary

Bristol, England

Interest in the relationship between diet and bile salt metabolism is logical since the admixture in the gut of food and the circulating bile salt pool, in a real sense, is an interaction of the environment with the organism. Specifically, it is the exposure to an important environmental variable of substances which, on return to the liver, are able to modify liver metabolism profoundly. Fiber could well be the most important of all the food components in this respect because it traverses the entire gut. In particular, it influences the function of the colon, which is the organ wherein bile salts are degraded by bacteria to substances with very different properties.

DIETARY FIBER

It should be stressed that fiber itself is not an article of diet. There are fiber-containing foods, fiber-lacking foods and fiber-depleted foods. Fiber-containing foods are simply all unprocessed plant products. Fiber-lacking foods are animal products, which are naturally free of fiber; whereas fiber-depleted foods are refined plant products that have been stripped of fiber by various mechanical processes. Fiber-depleted foods are artefacts of civilization. They should be divided into those that are totally depleted of fiber, notably the sugars and syrups, and those that are partly depleted, of which white flour in Western countries, is the main example. It is important to realize that in Western countries most of the carbohydrate eaten is refined, fiber-depleted carbohydrate.

DIETARY FIBER AND BILE SALT METABOLISM

In the field of bile salt metabolism there is a considerable amount of documented evidence for a relationship with dietary fiber. This evidence falls into four categories. The most informative and the most significant are those studies that have shown differences in bile salt metabolism between animals eating fiber-depleted diets and those eating natural diets. More specific, but harder to interpret, are studies that have shown the effects of feeding fiber-rich fractions of food such as bran. More specific yet, but more arbitrary and artificial and therefore more difficult to interpret, are studies wherein purified components of fiber are fed--cellulose, hemicellulose and so-called lignin, for example. And finally, there are the in vitro interactions of which Dr. Eastwood already has spoken.

Turning then to the differences in bile salt metabolism on fiber-depleted and natural diets, let me refer briefly to the experimental production of cholesterol-rich gallstones in animals. It is true that the pathogenesis of cholesterol gallstones and even of cholesterol precipitation is not fully developed, but it is generally agreed that disordered bile salt metabolism plays a prominent part. For this reason, it is relevant to draw your attention to the following fact. To my knowledge, diets that have been used to produce cholesterol gallstones in animals have been "semi-synthetic" diets. The point to be emphasized is that these "semi-synthetic" diets invariably are rich in fiber-depleted sugars or starches.

TABLE 1. Semi-Synthetic Diets Used to Produce Cholesterol-Rich Gallstones in Animals

Animal	Carbohydrates in Diet	Experimenters
Hamster	72% glucose or sucrose	Dam & Christensen (1952)
		Hikasa, et al. (1969)
Mouse	51% glucose	Tepperman, et al. (1964)
Prairie dog	34% sucrose, 14% cornstarch	Brenneman, et al. (1972)
Rabbit	7% sucrose, 6½% glucose, 6% cornstarch	Borgman & Haselden (1968)
Squirrel monkey	62% sucrose	Osuga & Portman (1971)
Dog	50% sucrose, 26% cornstarch	Englert, et al. (1969)

(from Bloomfield, 1963)

The accompanying table (Table 1) shows the main animal models that have been used to produce such gallstones, and the carbohydrates present in the diets (Bloomfield, 1963). In all instances, there is a high proportion (on the average 56%) of fiber-depleted sugar or starch in the diet. All the species listed in the table, except the dog, normally live on vegetable and plant foods, so they presumably are adapted to eating large amounts of carbohydrates. Therefore, if the pathogenic factor in these diets is the carbohydrate, and there is no convincing reason to implicate any other factor, then it must be not the amount but the type of carbohydrate. By type, I do not mean sugars as opposed to starch or simple as opposed to complex sugar (which is the usual division of carbohydrates), but rather the type in respect to fiber content.

The distinction here is between fiber-intact or natural carbohydrate and fiber-depleted carbohydrate. In animals, fiber-depleted or refined carbohydrate seems to be an essential component of a gallstone-producing diet. This suggests that bile salt metabolism may be influenced by dietary fiber.

Several studies have been made to compare bile salt metabolism in animals on semi-synthetic (fiber-depleted) diets and animals on natural diets rich in fiber. In rats, for example, diets containing 54-68% of sucrose or starch have been found repeatedly to reduce the fecal excretion of bile salts. Similarly, in rabbits this type of diet halved the fecal excretion of deoxycholate, which is the main bile salt in the rabbit. In monkeys, a semi-synthetic diet rich in carbohydrate but virtually free of fat was found by Redinger and his colleagues to reduce bile salt synthesis by two-thirds (Redinger, et al., 1973). The overall message from these varied studies is surely that fiber-depleted diets inhibit bile salt turnover or snythesis.

This point is illustrated in Figure 1 which shows that as fecal weight decreases so does the fecal bile acid excretion. In general, bile salt turnover is assessed by measuring either fecal excretion or hepatic synthesis. In the steady state these two must be equal, so that when there is reduced fecal excretion there also must be reduced synthesis of bile acids. Which comes first, reduced synthesis or reduced excretion on a fiber-depleted diet?

It is commonly assumed that reduced excretion is the initial or prime factor. This assumption arose because feeding very large amounts of purified cellulose has been shown to increase fecal bile salts. Feeding Metamucil® in rather more physiological doses accelerates the excretion of ^{14}C-labeled cholate, while in vitro fiber has bile salt binding properties. However, this assumption is not upheld by studies in which human volunteers have been fed a fiber-rich fraction of food, wheat bran. These observations

suggest rather that the primary action of fiber may be on the
liver.

STUDIES ON BRAN

Studies on bran have been carried out in Bristol by our group
and in Edinburgh by Eastwood's group. We have used ordinary
miller's bran which, according to Southgate, is approximately 6%
cellulose, 24% hemicelluloses and 4% lignin, but it is not a
highly standardized product (Southgate, 1969).

We first examined the effects of bran upon the production of
secondary bile salts. This was done by following the transfer of
a radioactive label from a primary bile salt to its dehydroxylated
derivatives in the bile. The method was to label the cholate pool
by injecting radioactive taurocholate, to collect bile from the

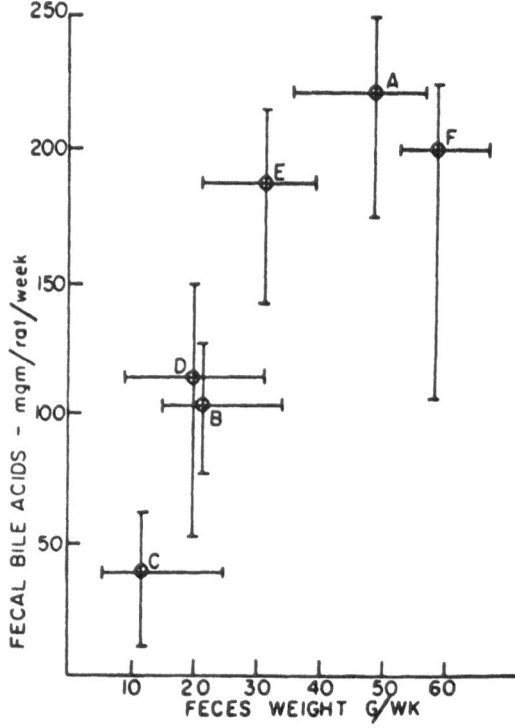

Fig. 1. Correlation between fecal bile acids and fecal weight
(mean ± S.D.) in rats on six different diets. The low-residue
diets B, D and E were semi-synthetic, while the others were based
on natural foods. Bile acid excretion was reduced on the semi-
synthetic diets (from Bloomfield, 1963).

duodenum on four successive mornings, to separate the bile salts, and then measure the radioactivity in the deoxycholate fractions. Figure 2 shows our results for five subjects whose gallbladders had been shown to function normally on cholecystography. When bran was added to the diet of these subjects in amounts of about 33 g a day the rate at which radioactivity appeared in deoxycholate in the bile was much reduced and this decline was significant statistically. We deduced that bran was altering bile salt metabolism in the colon because this is where dehydroxylation is believed to take place.

There are at least three possible explanations for these findings. First, less of the labeled taurocholate may have reached the colon with bran feeding. This implies that there is more efficient absorption in the ileum and seems unlikely. Second, dehydroxylation may have been prevented by a reduction in the number of anaerobic bacteria or in their dehydroxylating capacity. And third, absorption of deoxycholate may have been prevented. Our data do not enable us to decide which of these mechanisms is operating, but regardless, bran had distinctive effects on the composition of the bile salt pool.

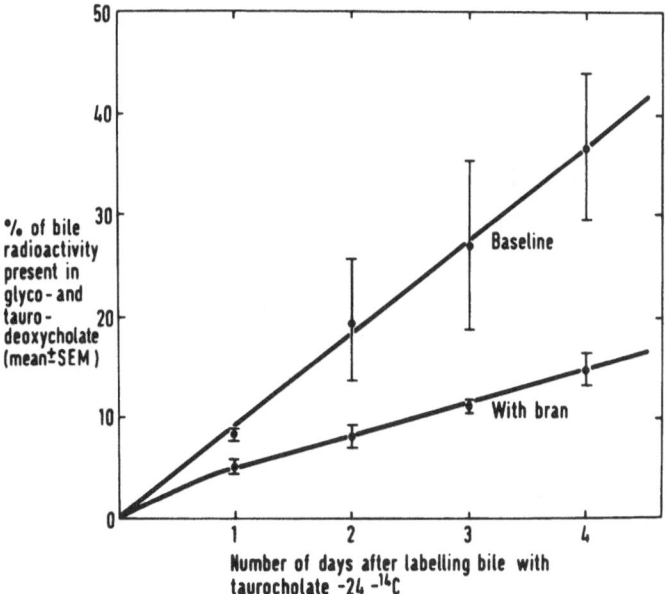

Fig. 2. The appearance of radioactivity in the conjugated deoxycholates in bile after administration of taurocholate 24-^{14}C. Results are shown for five subjects (mean ± S.E.) studied without and with the addition of bran to their normal diet.

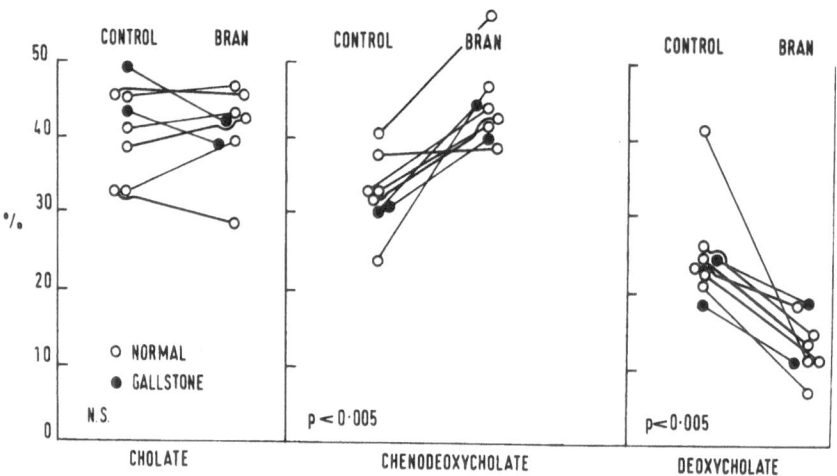

Fig. 3.   Composition of the bile salt pool expressed as percentages
of its three main components, cholate, chenodeoxycholate and
deoxycholate. Results in eight subjects before and after adding to
their diet bran 20-100 g/day (median 50 g).

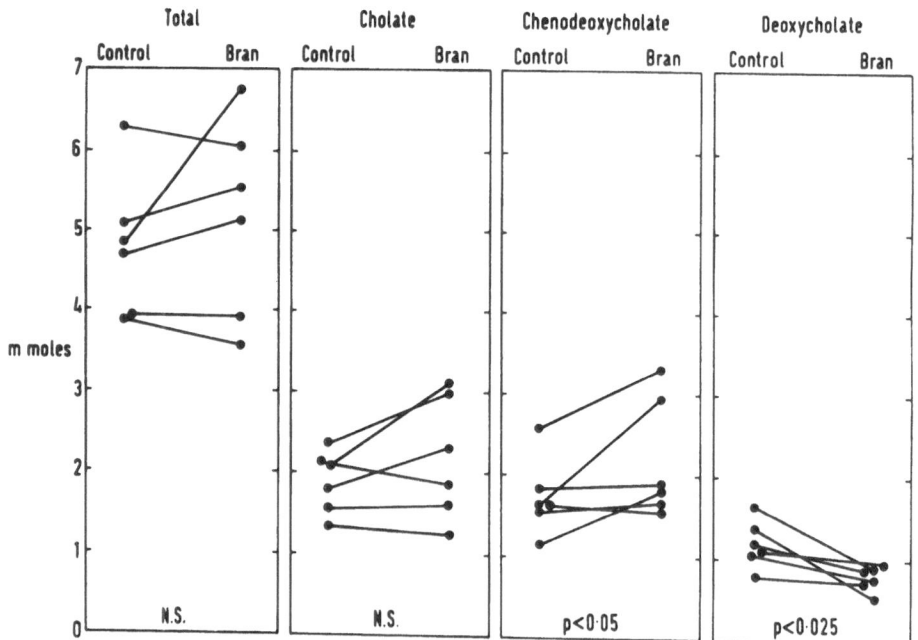

Fig. 4.   Size of the component and total bile salt pools in six
subjects before and during the administration of bran (mean
57 g/day, taken four to six weeks).

As shown in Figure 3, the effect of bran invariably was to
reduce the amount of deoxycholate in the bile to approximately
half its previous value. Unexpectedly, this was compensated for,
not by an increase in the precursor of deoxycholate, which is
cholate, but by an increase in chenodeoxycholate, which has no
known metabolic relationship with deoxycholate.

What is the significance of these changes? Presumably they
reflect changes in the pool sizes and production rates of the
different bile salts. Very recently we have been able to confirm
this finding by using the isotope dilution method after administration of cholate and chenodeoxycholate labeled with ^{14}C.
Figure 4 shows that the deoxycholate pool does decrease significantly while the chenodeoxycholate pool increases. As expected,
the cholate pool does not change.

The total bile salt pool also remains the same. I would like
to stress that after bran the deoxycholate pool always was less
than 1 millimole; whereas before bran, in all but one case, it was
more than 1 millimole. Why does the chenodeoxycholate pool
increase? The explanation comes from some parallel studies done
by Low-Beer and Pomare in Bristol on the effects of feeding
deoxycholate (Low-Beer & Pomare, 1973). They found that feeding
deoxycholate for two weeks caused a marked expansion of the
deoxycholate pool (which would be expected) and an equally dramatic
decrease in the chenodeoxycholate pool, but no change in the
cholate pool or the total bile salt pool. The decrease in the
chenodeoxycholate pool was associated with, and presumably caused
by, a decrease in the synthesis of chenodeoxycholate.

These exciting findings show that deoxycholate, which is a
secondary or colonic bile salt, exerts feedback inhibition on the
synthesis of one primary bile salt, chenodeoxycholate, but not on
the other one, cholate. This being so, it seems reasonable to
postulate that bran has the following effects upon bile salt
metabolism: Because less deoxycholate is absorbed from the colon
there is a smaller deoxycholate pool circulating to the liver.
This means that there is less inhibition of chenodeoxycholate
synthesis, which therefore increases, and the pool of chenodeoxycholate expands. Figure 5 shows that chenodeoxycholate synthesis
was indeed significantly increased by feeding bran, whereas
cholate synthesis was unaffected. Total bile salt synthesis tended
to increase, but by the paired "t" test the change was not significant.

CLINICAL IMPLICATIONS

Do these effects of bran have any clinical significance?
Here of course, one must speculate. However, there are reasons to

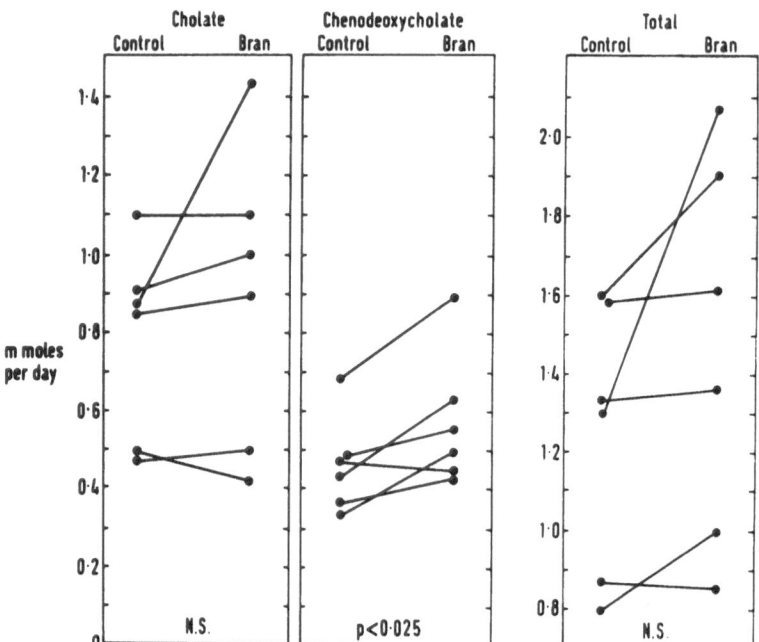

Fig. 5. Synthesis of the primary bile salts measured by isotope dilution in six subjects before and during the administration of bran.

suspect that changes in the relative amounts of deoxycholate and chenodeoxycholate in the bile may have important effects on lipid metabolism. This belief arises from the results of feeding deoxycholate and bran on the lipid composition of bile. Low-Beer and Pomare have found that the molar percentage of cholesterol in the bile, which is a fair estimate of the saturation of the bile with cholesterol, is significantly increased by feeding deoxycholic acid. Conversely, we have found recently that bran reduces the cholesterol saturation of bile, at least in patients with gallstones (Figure 6). We have not seen this effect of bran in normal subjects.

It appears, therefore, that feeding bran and feeding deoxycholate have "mirror image" effects on the bile. The size of the total bile salt pool does not change with either. With deoxycholate, bile becomes more saturated in cholesterol; while with bran it seems to become less saturated with cholesterol. At the same time, deoxycholate and bran have opposite effects on the composition of the pool, with deoxycholate decreasing and bran increasing the amount of chenodeoxycholate in circulation.

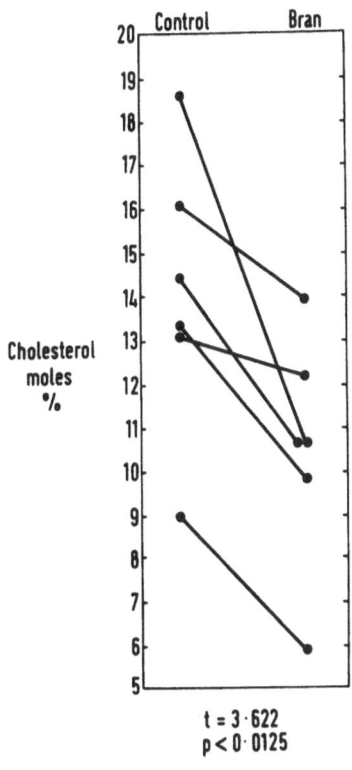

Fig. 6. Effect of feeding bran
(median 33g/day for four to five
weeks) on the molar concentration
of cholesterol in duodenal bile
of six subjects with radiolucent
stones in functioning gallbladders.
The data are expressed as the percentage of cholesterol in the
total lipid mixture of cholesterol,
phospholipids and bile salts.

Chenodeoxycholate is a bile salt with very special properties.
It is well known that feeding chenodeoxycholate dissolves gallstones by making the bile undersaturated with cholesterol. Simultaneously, it expands the chenodeoxycholate pool, but the total
bile salt pool is not always increased. The latest data suggest
that chenodeoxycholate works by suppressing the secretion of
cholesterol and not primarily by affecting bile salt secretion.
This raises the possibility that the secretion of cholesterol into
bile is normally regulated by the amount of chenodeoxycholate in
the bile salt pool, and this situation in turn could be determined
by the fiber content of the diet.

There are remarkable similarities between the actions of bran
and chenodeoxycholic acid. Both increase the chenodeoxycholate
pool and decrease the deoxycholate pool, and both decrease the
saturation of bile with cholesterol. There is one more similarity
and that is their effect on the fasting plasma triglyceride level.

Recent publications from the Hammersmith Hospital and the Mayo
Clinic have shown that feeding chenodeoxycholic acid significantly
reduces the plasma triglyceride level. In Bristol, we have measured

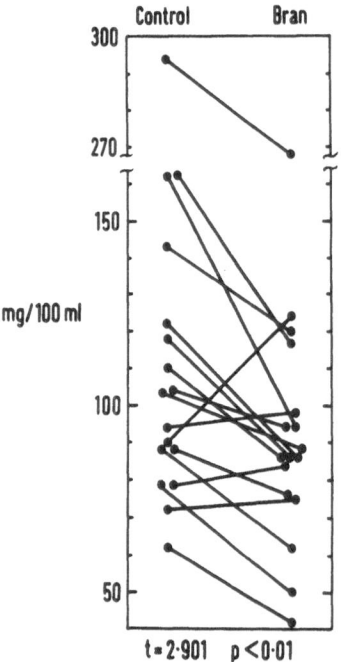

Fig. 7. Effect of feeding bran
(median 42 g/day for four to six
weeks) on plasma triglycerides of
17 subjects.

the plasma triglyceride levesl in 17 subjects before and after
adding bran to their diets for about five weeks and have noticed
a significant reduction of plasma triglycerides. (Figure 7) This
reduction occurred in all of the nine subjects whose levels were
above 100 mg per 100 ml initially.

    This effect of bran and of chenodeoxycholic acid on the blood
fits well with their effect on the bile. As Sodhi and Kudchodkar
have shown, the plasma triglyceride level correlates extremely well
with the rate of turnover of cholesterol, as measured by various
means such as isotope kinetics. Secretion into bile probably is
the chief pathway for the excretion of cholesterol. Therefore, a
fall in cholesterol turnover should be evidenced by a fall in both
bile cholesterol secretion and plasma triglycerides. This being
so, it seems probable that both chenodeoxycholic acid and bran
reduce cholesterol turnover. This in turn raises the possibility
that dietary fiber may be a natural controller of cholesterol
production.

    In conclusion, I apologize for the preliminary nature of some
of my data and for the largely speculative element in my deductions.
I can only plead that this meeting was designed more to frame
questions than to provide neatly fitted answers; and I hope I have
indicated at least a few questions that we can try to answer and
ideas that we can begin to test.

REFERENCES

Bloomfield, D. K., 1963, Dynamics of cholesterol metabolism
    I. Factors regulating total sterol biosynthesis and accumu-
    lation in the rat, Proc. Nat. Acad. Sci., U.S.A., $\underline{50}$:117-124.

Low-Beer, T. S., Pomare, E. W., 1973, The human bile salt feedback
    mechanism and its specificity, Gastroenterology, $\underline{64}$:764.

Redinger, R. N., Hermann, A. H., Small, D. M., 1973, Primate bilary
    physiology X. Effects of diet and fasting on biliary lipid
    secretion and relative compositions and bile salt metabolism
    in the Rhesus monkey, Gastroenterology, $\underline{64}$:610-621.

Southgate, D. A. T., 1969, Determination of carbohydrates in foods.
    II. Unavailable carbohydrates, J. Sci. Food Agric., $\underline{20}$:331-335.

DISCUSSION

M. A. Eastwood: Dr. Heaton, in fact, is measuring a different
phenomenon from that which we are measuring with fecal bile acids.
Certainly, we find that bran does not alter the amount of deoxycholic acid in the stool. On the other hand, when we tried the
effect of bran on fecal bile acids, it was in the control period
after bran feeding that the total fecal bile acids began to rise
quite markedly, although there was no qualitative change. Whether
this is a delayed effect or whether we did not give bran for long
enough, I do not know. It seems possible that there may be two
pools or two phases of bile acid; one is a fast phase which is the
duodenal-ileal cycle, and the other may be a colonic phase which
is much slower in its dynamics.

K. W. Heaton: I do not think there is any evidence that deoxycholate is formed anywhere or absorbed anywhere except in the
colon; and since our data indicate that something is happening to
deoxycholate, then bran must be doing something in the colon.

I. H. Rosenberg: Previous experiments on iliectomy patients
in a number of laboratories have shown changes that are very similar
to the changes you have just described with bran feeding. Presumably an increased turnover leads to a decreased amount of deoxycholate and an increased amount of chenodeoxycholic acid. I wonder
if the mechanism is not, at least in part, interruption of the
enterohepatic circulation? To what extent do you see another evidence of this action? As chenodeoxy synthesis rises, is there a
shift of the glycine/taurine ratio?

K. W. Heaton: Yes. Although we began with the expectation
of showing that bran reduces the absorption of bile acids and, in
a sense, performs a mini-iliectomy, our data in fact have not shown
this, because the half-life of the labeled bile acids is not influenced by feeding bran. The G/T ratio, as I recollect, rises slightly
but not significantly.

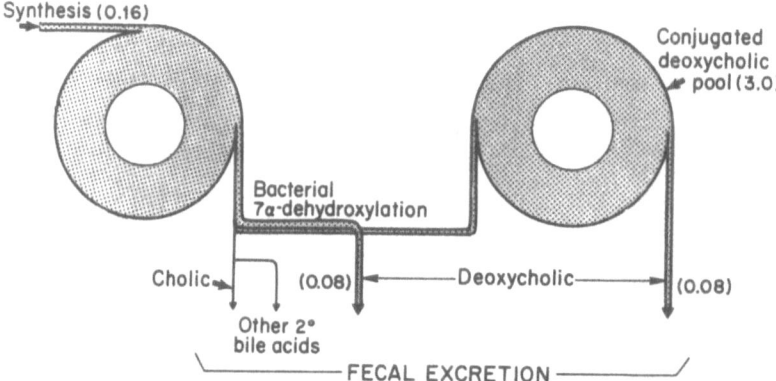

Fig. 1. Enterohepatic circulation of cholic acid (left) and deoxycholic acid (right). The horizontal tangent at upper left
(synthesis) represents de novo synthesis of cholic acid from cholesterol. Efficient intestinal conservation results in the formation of a cholic acid pool (left annulus). Cholic acid that is
lost from enterohepatic circulation is 7α-hydroxylated to form
deoxycholic acid, part of which is excreted (center arrow) and part
of which is absorbed. The absorbed deoxycholic acid passes to the
liver, where it is conjugated. The deoxycholic acid conjugates are
efficiently conserved, resulting in the formation of a deoxycholic
acid pool (right annulus). The deoxycholic acid lost from the
enterohepatic circulation (vertical tangent, lower right) is balanced by new input from the colon.

A. F. Hofmann: I would like to introduce some figures that
conceivably might unite the apparently conflicting points of view
of Drs. Eastwood and Heaton. Figure 1 is Dr. Heaton's ring and,
as he mentioned, the cholic acid is conjugated and recycled, the
free cholate returning for reconjugation. In the colon we have 7-
alpha-dehydroxylation forming deoxycholic acid and some fraction of

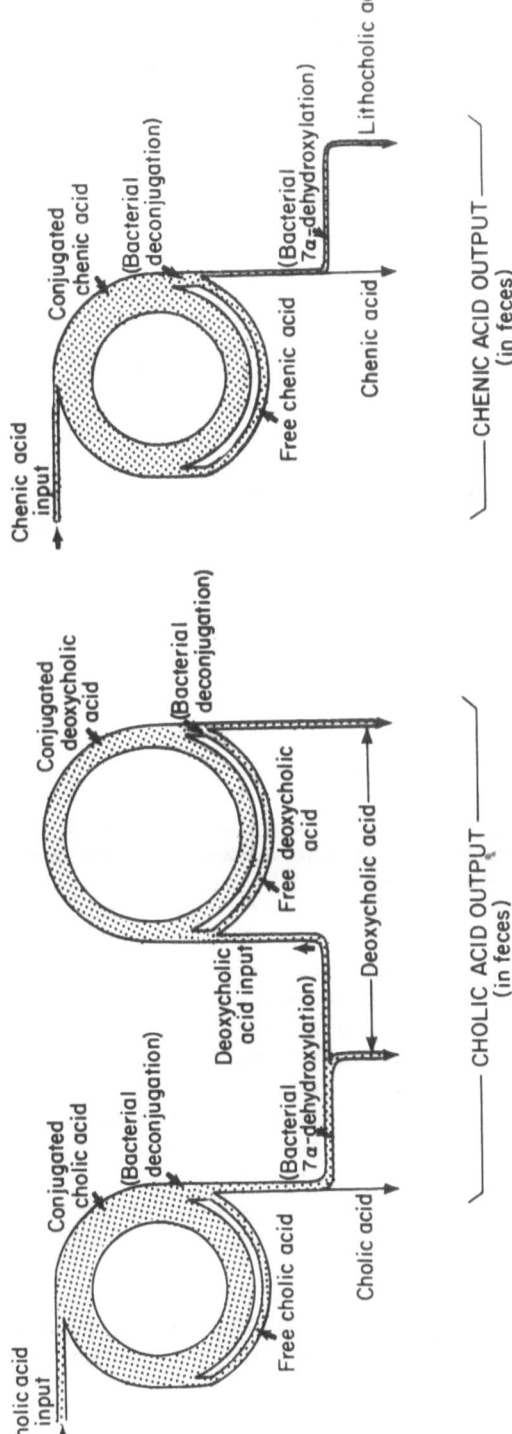

Fig. 2. (Left) Enterohepatic circulation of cholic acid and deoxycholic acid; for explanation, see Figure 1. (Right) Enterohepatic circulation of chenodeoxycholic (chenic) acid; enterohepatic circulation of lithocholate is not shown. If dietary fiber decreases deoxycholic acid input, then intestinal conservation of chenic acid may increase, so that for a given chenic acid input, chenic acid pool is larger. The results will be an increased proportion of chenic acid in bile.

the deoxycholic acid that is made is reabsorbed. This returns to
the liver and is secreted in bile, to be conserved by reabsorption
in the small intestine. This is how the deoxycholic acid pool
arises. The deoxycholic output is balanced by the deoxycholic acid
input. The easiest way to explain Dr. Heaton's data is that bran
decreases the deoxycholic input. Therefore Dr. Eastwood, in looking at fecal deoxycholic acid, should detect no difference. Normally the fraction of deoxycholic acid which is absorbed is about
one-third to one-half. If this fraction decreases to one-fifth,
the deoxycholic acid pool would get smaller.

Figure 2 shows the three major bile acids: cholic, deoxycholic
and chenodeoxycholic. If the deoxycholic pool decreases and chenodeoxycholic synthesis increases, then the chenodeoxycholic acid pool
will be enriched. In addition, deoxycholic and chenodeoxycholic
acid may compete for small intestinal conservation. If so, when
deoxycholic acid input decreases, the chenodeoxycholic acid pool
will expand even for the same degree of synthesis. Thus, if synthesis goes up and intestinal conservation increases, the chenodeoxycholic acid pool will respond exactly as Dr. Heaton has
observed. I believe, therefore, that we can explain this apparent
difference on a fairly rational basis.

G. J. Devroede: We seem to imply, if an event occurs when bran
is fed, that bran is causing this event and I think that we have a
problem of correlation. For instance, the output of bile acids
into the duodenum in response to pancreozymin was less in healthy
subjects fed an elemental diet (Flexical,[R] Mead-Johnson), than in
those taking the control diet (Figure 3). The difference between
these diets is not in the carbohydrate fraction, but in the fact
that the casein is hydrolyzed in the elemental diet and part of the
long-chain triglycerides is replaced by medium-chain triglycerides.

Two things may correlate for one of four reasons: one causes
the other and that is the conclusion we accept most readily; they
may correlate because they are caused by a common factor (as, for
example there is in New York City a correlation of 0.96 between
neonatal death and ice cream consumption, because both rise with
heat). There may be a causal interrelationship and interdependency,
for instance, between migraine headache and irritability (one does
not necessarily cause the other); and the fourth possibility is
that this may be pure chance (for instance, there is a correlation
between the length of dresses in England and the amount of rainfall
in India).

A. F. Hofmann: No one here would dispute what you say, Dr.
Devroede, in its philosophical scope, but science is concerned with
defining mechanisms in more detail in order to establish causality

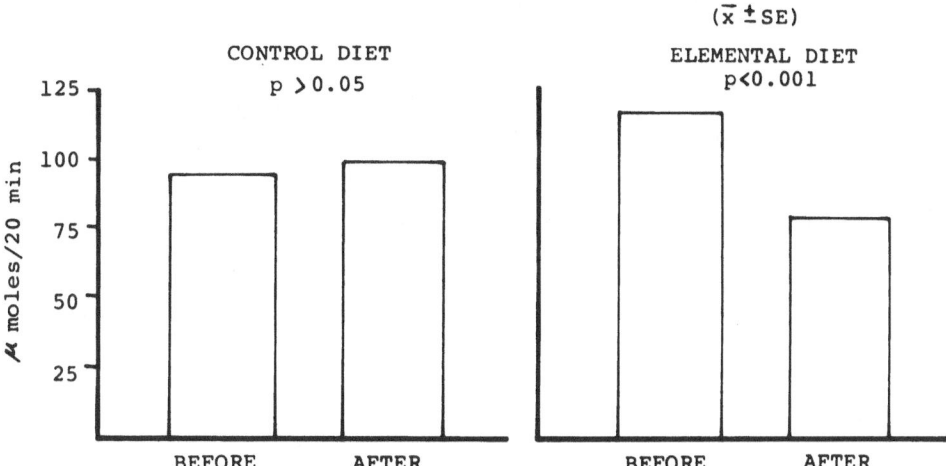

Fig. 3. Effect of an elemental diet on quantitative output of bile salts in the duodenum of healthy subjects after pancreozymin stimulation.

in the best traditions of David Hume. I think that Dr. Heaton has developed a logical scheme.

S. F. Phillips: I am impressed by variations in the composition and in the physiological effects of fiber from different plants and even from the same plant of different ages. How uniform is fiber composition and, therefore, how confident can one be as to the physiologic effects of the various brans? Has this question been examined? Can we assume that the bran fed in Bristol is the same as that employed in Edinburgh?

K. W. Heaton: This is only one of many questions Dr. Phillips, and there are no data on that point. We now are simply at the stage of discovering that a phenomenon exists. The next stage is to find out under what circumstances it occurs; to plot dose-response curves; to identify modifying factors, and so on. I agree with you that bran is not a well-standardized product. We obviously made sure that all our subjects took the same kind of bran, but in England there are two very different varieties on sale; one, powdery and the other, flaky. I can well believe that

they have different effects; they are, in fact, made in slightly
different ways.

S. F. Phillips: Is the problem important enough to demand
the use of a uniform product even if we do not know its exact composition or the physiological effects?

K. W. Heaton: Yes, I think it is.

A. F. Hofmann: In fact, Dr. Heaton, would it not be more
accurate if your papers were entitled the effect of miller's bran
rather than the effect of dietary fiber?

K. W. Heaton: I think the word "bran" has usually appeared
in the title.

H. M. Spiro: Would you say that bran has an exclusively
beneficent effect as compared with other fiber, or have you used
bran simply because it is convenient?

K. W. Heaton: The reason we chose bran was because it is a
convenient and very concentrated way of obtaining fiber. It is 89%
solid matter. If we had carried out these experiments by feeding
carrots, I don't think the volunteers would have remained volunteers
very long. Dr. Eastwood probably could make his calculation more
quickly that I can, but I imagine it would have involved eating six
or eight pounds of carrots a day.

A. F. Hofmann: No, but the message is that although this kind
of bran has a very interesting effect, we do not know about the
effects of other brans.

M. A. Eastwood: It is evidently important that we should consider fiber from all sources. I do not think there is anything
exclusive about wheat bran. At the moment, we have an experiment
in progress repeating the work done with bran, but using dried
carrots. The observed effects are greater than those noted with
bran. We have made a clinical comparison of bran of a coarse nature
with bran resembling flour in appearance. The coarser bran is much
more effective in reducing colonic pressure than is the floury bran.
It obviously is necessary to define the physical characteristics,
the type and the variety of the fiber source.

A. F. Hofmann: Then at this point it is impossible to state
dogmatically that all brans will work or that certain brans will
not work.

M. A. Eastwood: That's right. The only thing that we have is
a variety of vegetable dietary sources which we can grade in order

of their capacity to swell. It would appear that carrots, bran,
apples and oranges are far superior in terms of their potential to
increase stool weight than are cauliflower and potatoes.

A. F. Hofmann: But your swelling studies have been done before they pass through the small intestine where they may be
totally modified. Your data may be totally irrelevant. Isn't that
correct?

M. A. Eastwood: The swelling studies were done on fiber from
which the liquids and protein had been removed. So far as I know
there is no modification in the small intestine of the polysaccharides which swell. The modifications take place in the colon.

A. M. Connell: I think one other necessary control is the
nature of the subject under study. Encouraged by some preliminary
results showing lower serum triglycerides and serum cholesterols
in people with various hyperlipedemias, we have subjected about
half of our second-year medical school class, who for the most part
are healthy, to eating bran. These are diets that are carefully
controlled as to calorie consumption. After two months, there is
no difference at all between those who have this dietary supplement
and those who do not. So I suspect that we are dealing with different groups of people. I would be interested in your comment on
your triglyceride study in that it appeared to demonstrate that
only those who had high levels initially showed the greatest
decrease.

K. W. Heaton: The subjects were all middle-aged and nearly
all women. I think the middle-aged aspect might be important
because, as you know, triglycerides tend to rise with age and what
we are trying to do in these experiments is to lower an elevated
substance. Therefore, if you take young men whose triglycerides
have not yet started to rise, it may not be possible to show any
effect.

A. M. Connell: I think this is the point.

K. W. Heaton: Yes, I agree.

M. M. Stanley: These are very exciting observations. They
will significantly influence our own future studies. I have had
the same experience in trying to get experimental subjects to take
large quantities of these inert materials. I am amazed that
Shurpalekar could motivate his Indian children to take 100 g of
cellulose a day. I have had great difficulty in administering 30 g
a day. In the U.S.A. bran cereal has enjoyed a modest popularity
but it is usually taken at breakfast. Could your results be repro-
duced with the same amount of material taken once a day rather than

three times day? Again, in one of your recent papers with Pomare
(Pomare and Heaton, 1973) you reported that bran feeding in subjects with an intact gallbladder inhibited 7-alpha-dehydroxylation.
This promoted excessive deconjugation of cholyl taurine (taurocholate). Can you explain this effect?

K. W. Heaton: I was very puzzled by it until I discussed it
with Dr. Hofmann yesterday. He made the reasonable suggestion,
that the effect of bran is to force the bile salt pool farther down
the small intestine before it is absorbed and therefore into an
area, namely the terminal ileum, which is richer in deconjugating
bacteria. It is known that up to 100% deconjugation can take place
in the terminal ileum. I do not know if Dr. Eastwood would agree
that this would fit with his studies in rats. Does the bile salt
pool tend to move further down the intestine on a higher fiber intake?

M. A. Eastwood: It is not possible to alter the distribution
of bile acids along the small intestine, i.e., principally in the
ileum, but the rat of course does not have a gallbladder, so it is
a very special case. We do not know whether it is analogous to the
cholecystectomized human.

K. W. Heaton: Yes. It is of interest, incidentally, that bran
does not seem to have the effects which I described to you in cholecystectomized individuals.

M. A. Stanley: The diets often eaten by Europeans and
Americans have been termed "fiber-deficient." These and other diets
also may be relatively deficient in other nutrients such as calcium,
zinc and iron. Further, the fiber deficiency actually may compen-
sate for the deficient intake of calcium, etc. Thus, when bran
alone, or other fiber constituents are added to some of the diets,
the consequently increased fecal excretion of calcium and zinc
actually may result in a negative balance (Rheinhold, et al., 1973)
so that if we're going to replace a "fiber deficiency" alone, then
we are creating another problem. Moreover by adding bran, whether
we call it replacing a deficiency or not, we are producing another
"mal-absorption syndrome." I think you demonstrated this effect in
the increased fecal excretion of nitrogen and fat.

A. F. Hofmann: Does fiber increase fecal fat?

K. W. Heaton: Dr. Southgate showed that fecal fat can be
increased up to 8 g a day.

M. A. Stanley: Eight or nine g a day. This is not usually
shown on the insensitive balance studies commonly done, but it can
be shown with indicator studies. An increase of up to 100 to 150%

in fecal fat and nitrogen is produced by various of these fiber supplements.

A. F. Hofmann: Is that bad, Dr. Stanley?

M. M. Stanley: No, I do not say it is bad, but by definition it is either malabsorption or increased fecal excretion from endogenous sources. I am not certain of the pathogenesis nor the source of these materials that are excreted in excess. They may originate in the colon from increased desquamation of epithelial cells or from other processes. If not endogenous, they may be consequent to an effect of bran in reducing normal absorption of usual dietary protein and fat. This probably occurs with calcium, zinc and iron (ref. cited) but is less likely for protein and fat. Finally, a third possibility is that these fecal residues originate in bran from "unavailable" constituents (Southgate and Durnin, 1970; James and Cummings, 1974). If so, this would ordinarily be categorized as "malabsorption"; perhaps "controlled malabsorption" would be an appropriate term.

Similarly, these bran components may be more "available" to certain colonic organisms than to the host. Certainly the observed effects of bran upon bowel function are often the direct and indirect consequences of changes induced in colonic flora.

J. H. Cummings: It is true that adding bran to the diet increases fecal fat. In what I hope are fairly well controlled metabolic studies, fecal fat increases from a mean of 20.45g/week (± 4.7 S.D.) to 30.43g/week (± 3.9 S.D.) on adding cereal fiber to the diet.

A. F. Hofmann: There is no fat in the bran, is there?

J. H. Cummings: Yes, bran contains about 4% fat, nearly all in the form of polyunsaturated fatty acids. A proportion of these fatty acids are covalently linked to the various fibers in the bran and therefore we think they are relatively unavailable to the normal digestive processes of the small intestine. If the fecal fatty acid composition is examined by gas chromatography in people on high fiber diets, a number of unusual fatty acids appear. These fatty acids probably are omega-hydroxy-fatty acids and they account for part of the increase in the fecal fat in these subjects. There are other fatty acids in bran itself which are "available" and these probably are absorbed.

A. F. Hofmann: So in part you are saying that the apparent malabsorption as defined by Dr. Stanley is artefactual and is related to covalently linked fatty acids in the bran. These then are released by either bacterial lipases or alkaline saponification in the routine determination of fecal fat. Is that correct?

J. H. Cummings: Yes, that's right.

A. F. Hofmann: Presumably they would be released by lipases because we do not think that the bacterial hydrases which make hydroxy fatty acids could probably operate on covalently linked fatty acids. Presumably step one is bacterial lipolysis and step two is a bacterial formation of hydroxy fatty acids. Is that your interpretation?

J. H. Cummings: Not exactly. In fact, the bran itself contains hydroxy fatty acid which is normally present in the waxes and in the cuticles of plants. Plant wax itself is a complex polymer of hydroxy fatty acids and other fatty acids and it seems unlikely that any normal digestive enzyme attacks them. They are therefore excreted and then hydrolyzed during technics for measuring fats in the stools. Fecal nitrogen also increases on a high fiber diet and the same sort of argument can be applied.

J. H. Dietschy: I would like to discuss some of the interesting observations, and to suggest some fruitful lines for future work in relation to a number of recent advances in the fields of transport and bile acid and steroid metabolism.

The first observation, repeated here as well as in the literature, is that fibers, pectins, and a variety of plant substances, in some way alter the rate of absorption of a number of substrates. This suggests that they may alter bile acid metabolism, and that they may interfere with the absorption of cholesterol, water and electrolytes, and a variety of other substrates. It seems to me that we now are in a position to examine this situation in a much more sophisticated way because of the great increase in available background information on factors determining rates of absorption.

Basically the overall rate of absorption of any product or any substrate in the colon is determined by events in the bulk phase as well as in the phenomenon of membrane transport. That is, the membrane maintains the carrier mechanisms for active transport and it dictates the permeability co-efficients for passively absorbed substances, but the major determinants in many systems are those events occurring in the bulk solution, which is in this case, the gut contents. With a passively absorbed material, for example, the rate of absorption will be equal to the product: (the chemical activity of the particular ion or substance in question) times (the permeability coefficient which that molecule has for penetrating the membrane).

There is considerable recent evidence to suggest that the permeability characteristics of all membranes in the mammal are quite
similar. This may seem surprising, but nevertheless, it is so for
the seven mammalian membranes that have now been quantitated, so
that specificity of uptake probably depends, again, upon bulk phase
phenomena. To illustrate: If a passive bile acid absorption is
proceeding in the colon, and if bile acid is introduced in a very
dilute and simple solution, the rate of uptake is equal to the product of that chemical concentration or activity times its appropriate permeability co-efficient. If a binding agent or a micelle
of any type is introduced, thereby reducing the chemical activity,
the rate of uptake necessarily is reduced.

Now, despite the somewhat pessimistic view presented here on
the difficulties of working with these complicated materials, there
is an enormous industrial literature dealing with co-polymer physical chemistry, and these co-polymers behave very much like lectins,
or cellulose. I suspect that the same principles that apply to the
industrially-made polymers, which can be administered or used in a
variety of processes, apply also to various plant fibers.

These polymers can be built on a carbon backbone, on a cellulose backbone, on a variety of other backbones. By changing the
side groups, one can make these polymers ionic or non-ionic, hydrophobic or hydrophilic, and capable of adsorbing bacteria, viruses,
toxins, and various substrates with more or less specificity. It
is not surprising, therefore, that different kinds of fibers produce different effects.

It seems to me that the technics of physical chemistry could
now be used to examine the apparent isoelectric point of various
purified fibers, even after subjecting them to digestion and
recovery from the intestine of an animal. Such measurements might
help to determine if new kinds of products were being formed and
would provide at least an initial approach to the effects on binding and how the binding constants or the permeability factors might
be changed.

It seems likely that any changes in terms of gross absorption
of any product in the gut are not attributable to an effect upon
permeability co-efficients, but rather to an effect based upon the
physical state of substrate in the gut, i.e., a differential and
preferential binding by different compounds. With such techniques
as equilibrium dialysis and affinity chromatography, this problem
can be approached in a reasonable way that would make some sense
out of what is at present a very imprecise science.

The second aspect of this situation seems to be the important
relationship between these binding agents, these polymers, e.g.,

plant polymers, and bacterial metabolism. As I have indicated, one
can produce commercial polymers which preferentially and with high-
specificity bind certain viruses or certain bacteria. The important
question seems to be this: does a bacterium that is bound to a solid
surface (i.e., to a polymer) carry on metabolic functions in a normal way? Such a study might produce interesting data provided the
binding of the substrate could be factored. One would have to be
extraordinarily careful to discriminate from the parallel binding
of the substrate.

Again, there is a precedent for this approach in the biochemical literature dealing with enzyme kinetics in enzyme systems in
which there is fixation to matrices, where there are remarkable differences in the kinetics. This type of investigation could have
important implications in terms of changes, not merely in numbers
of bacteria, which is a relatively crude measurement even by the
best technics; but also of changes in the metabolic behavior of the
same number of bacteria bound to a fiber, or to a particle of some
sort of polymer.

The next point deals with the whole interaction of these various fiber compounds and various aspects of lipid metabolism. Some
of the implications disturb me. First, one should be extraordinarily
cautious about interpreting the data on serum lipids. I have
recently reviewed the research at some of the large lipid centers
in this country, where it has been shown that the degree of lowering of the serum triglycerides demonstrated at this meeting actually
is less than is manifested in most of the placebo groups. That is,
that small changes in cholesterol or triglyceride in an uncontrolled
group of patients in which the Hawthorne effect or placebo effect
enters in, are extremely difficult to interpret.

The remaining points deal with the interrelationship of chenodeoxycholic acid and cholesterol metabolism, and with the effects
of various changes in diet quality on these parameters. This whole
interrelationship is often put into the context of bile acid feedback on HMG Co-A reductase in the liver, which is the rate-limiting
enzyme in cholesterogenesis. It is unquestionable that bile acid
feeding shuts off HMG Co-A reductase, but that this is a bile acid
effect is very questionable. In fact, one can expand the bile acid
pool by three or four times, but if the absorption of cholesterol
into the circulation is eliminated by lymphatic diversion, there is
no inhibition of HMG Co-A reductase at all. Furthermore, the implication that feeding fiber somehow turns off hepatic cholesterogenesis requires much more supporting evidence than is now available.
Indeed, the experimental results suggest quite the opposite. In
the experimental animal, changing from a highly purified diet to a
fiber-containing diet actually increases cholesterogenesis three-
or four- or five-fold.

Finally, there is the other problem of whether or not bile acid feeding can modify bile acid synthesis. As Dr. Hofmann and others would agree, there must be feedback regulation, but this is currently a very confused field. I think the problem principally is that the assay now being used for 7-alpha-hydroxylation, which used labeled cholesterol as a substrate, contains a major artifact. As a result, many of the reported assays are seriously in error, as was recently reported from England.

Clearly, changes in the fiber content of the diet, either by direct or indirect mechanisms, probably have a striking effect upon the total steroid balance and this effect may be accomplished through the metabolism of bile acids, through binding or cholesterol, or through modification of micellar effects. These interrelationships are very poorly understood at present and we need to be cautious in interpreting the results.

REFERENCES

James, W. P. T., Cummings, J. H., 1974, Dietary fiber and energy regulation, Lancet, 1:61-62.

Pomare, E. W., Heaton, K. W., 1973, Alteration of bile salt metabolism by dietary fiber. Brit. Med. J., 4:262-264.

Rheinhold, J. G., Nasr, K., Lahimgarzadel, A., Hedayali, H., 1973, Effects of purified phytate and phytate-rich bread on metabolism of zinc, calcium, phosphorus and nitrogen in man, Lancet 1: 283-287.

Southgate, D. A. T., Durnin, J. V. G. A., 1970, Calorie conversion factors: An experimental re-assessment of the factors used in the calculation of the energy value of human diets, Brit. J. Nutr. 24:517-535.

PART II

FIBER AND COLONIC FUNCTION

ABSORPTION FROM THE HUMAN COLON

S. F. Phillips

The Mayo Clinic

Rochester, Minnesota

In approaching a study of absorption from the human colon, it is important to consider a spectrum of circumstances under which absorption across a membrane can be examined. At one end of the spectrum, a clean membrane can be established in vitro with an Ussing chamber having artificial, saline solutions on both sides of the membrane. At the other extreme, the colon in vivo functions in the presence of extremely heterogenous contents, an important difference to be taken into account in the interpretation and the application of experimental data to the human situation. We also must realize that any differences in gut function under different circumstances may be determined by the properties of the membrane itself or by the manner in which the organ functions in life. A second factor quite apart from membrane function, is the chemical nature of the gut contents, that is, the material in the lumen that will be absorbed. It already has been mentioned that the lumen of the colon contains a complex bacterial eco-system. These circumstances obviously affect the substrate that is available for absorption.

This subject can be considered under five sub-headings:
1) input to the colon; 2) actual membrane properties; 3) factors that modify membrane function; and some 4) chemical and 5) physical factors as they relate to absorptive function in vivo.

1. Input to the Colon. It has been traditional to assume that the material that comes out of an ileostomy is the same as that which goes into the colon in health. Table 1 shows the output of water and electrolytes from an established ileostomy. I draw attention to the volume, 400 to 700 ml per day. Sodium is the major cation. For comparison, the table also gives figures for the output of

TABLE 1.   Established Ileostomy Output

Author		24 Hour Output		
	Vol (ml)	Electrolytes (mEq)		
	Water	Sodium	Potassium	Chloride
Fowler (1959)		20-70	<10	
Smiddey (1960)		30-60	3-4	
Nuguid (1961)	600	45-90	5-15	15-30
Gallagher (1962)	690	85	5.0	
Kramer (1962)	466	60	3.6	
Kanaghinis (1963)	429	53	5.5	
		24 Hour Fecal Composition		
Berger (1960)	100	0.5-5	5-15	0.5-3

water and sodium in the normal stools. For reasons that do not
concern us now, there is little basis for the assumption that
equates ileostomy effluent and colonic input. I shall now describe
some studies that employed a different approach, namely an attempt
to quantify what goes through the terminal ileum and into the cecum
in a healthy subject.

Giller and I used a perfusion technic to quantify the volume
and composition of material entering the colon in health (Phillips
& Giller, 1973). We positioned a tube in the terminal ileum and
used a slow, constant infusion of marker solution to label the
intestinal contents. By aspirating the contents downstream from
our labeling site and by measuring marker dilution, the volume of
ileal content could be determined. We also gave our subjects a
fecal marker daily, and they ingested a standard diet for a period
of one to three weeks. The period of ileal sampling was 36 to 48
hours and fecal collections were made during a three-day period at
the end of the study. The results are shown in Figure 1. Estimated
ileal composition is shown on the left of each graph; composition
of the stools, collected under balanced conditions is shown on the
right. The data are from five healthy subjects; the shaded areas
indicate the ranges. The average input to the colon was 1500 ml
per day, or approximately twice the volume excreted by ileostomy
patients. Similarly, total colonic absorption in our studies was
about twice that estimated by comparing ileostomy and fecal losses.
To date, studies employing this technique have been directed only
towards water and electrolyte absorption.

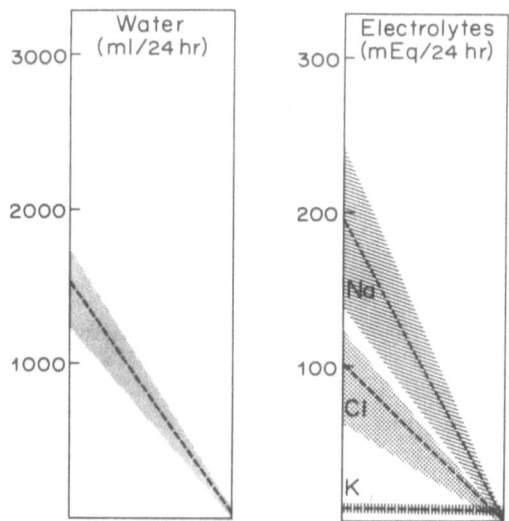

Fig. 1. Comparison of 24-hour ileal content and feces in health.

2. <u>Membrane Properties</u>. A standard technic for study of mucosal
function in colonic perfusion, first described by Levitan, et al.
(1962). A multi-lumen tube is passed into the cecum and proximal
aspiration sites can be used to remove ileal contents (Devroede &
Phillips, 1969). Test fluids are perfused into the cecum; the
fluid traverses the colon and is recovered through a rectal tube.
Steady-state perfusion conditions can be established relatively
easily, and absorption can be measured in the whole colon, relative
to nonabsorbable markers. Absorptive capacity for water per 24
hours in the healthy human colon has been extrapolated from perfusion studies. These methods show an average rate of water
absorption by the entire colon of 2 ml per minute which, when
extrapolated, yields approximately 3 liters a day. This figure is
similar to that we measured by a colonic input study in a patient
with sprue (Phillips & Giller, 1973). She had an input to the colon
of 3500 ml per 24 hours and a fecal volume of about 500 ml per day.

     Next, let us consider some aspects of electrolyte absorption.
Devroede and I (Devroede & Phillips, 1969) measured the absorption
of sodium and chloride when the colon was perfused with different
initial concentrations of saline (Figure 2). Luminal concentration
of sodium or chloride is on the abscissa and absorption is on the
ordinate. In all but one subject, sodium was absorbed when it was
infused at 25 meq per liter; absorption of sodium increased in a
linear fashion with concentration. Chloride absorption was even
more striking. When chloride was infused at 25 meq per liter, all

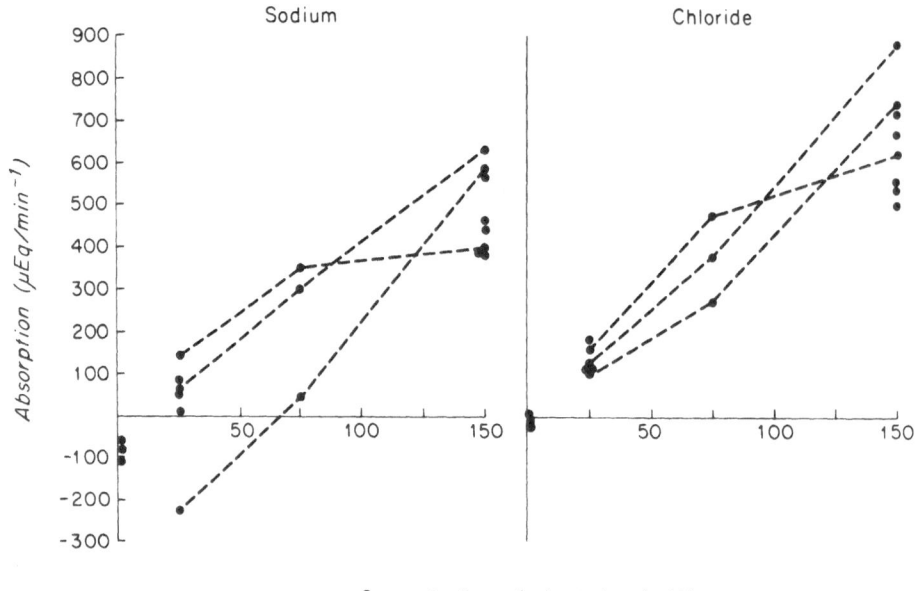

Fig. 2.   Absorption of electrolytes by human colon.

subjects absorbed significant amounts.   These and other studies
demonstrate very clearly that, per unit surface area, the membrane
of the colon is more efficient at absorbing sodium and chloride
than is any other part of the gastrointestinal tract.   In association
with chloride absorption, there always is secretion of bicarbonate,
i.e., there is a reciprocity between the movement of these two
anions.   Our studies indicate that significant amounts of potassium
move across the colonic mucosa by passive mechanisms.   There is a
high negative mucosal potential difference in the colon, approximately 40 to 50 mv, and this electrical force promotes, by simple
passive mechanisms, an accumulation of potassium in the lumen to
approximately two to three times its concentration in extracellular fluid.   As an additional factor, there is a component of
secretion that occurs by way of colonic mucus.   Colonic mucus has
a high concentration of potassium and mucus may represent a separate
pool, that is, a separate secretory pathway, for potassium in the
colon.

Is absorption different at various levels in the colon?
Devroede studied this using a) the perfusion technic, b) the rectum
isolated by a large balloon, and c) infusion studies at different
levels of the colon (Devroede, et al., 1971).   They found the
following differences: The maximum rate of water and sodium

absorption occurred in the cecum, and there was a descending
gradient of absorptive function from the cecum to the rectum
(Figure 3). We published some of these observations under the
title "Failure of the rectum to absorb sodium and water". Two
other groups have shown subsequently that we overstated the case.
The differences are more matters of degree; absorption in the
rectum is significantly slower than that in the colon and the left
colon absorbs more slowly than the right colon.

What other materials are absorbed from the colon? These
observations come largely from perfusion studies and are rather
fragmentary (Table 2). When the colon is perfused with fatty
acid, oleic acid and ricinoleic acid are absorbed. Medium-chain
fatty acids also are absorbed in man. Bile acid absorption has
been measured in some studies. Mekhjian (Mekhjian, et al., 1971)
in our laboratory observed appreciable absorption of unconjugated
bile acids in the clean perfused human colon, apparently by a
passive mechanism. We have few data on the absorption of other
materials in man. In animal studies, glucose and amino acids are
absorbed from the colon by passive diffusion. I shall not deal
with short-chain fatty acid absorption because Dr. Levitt will
mention this later.

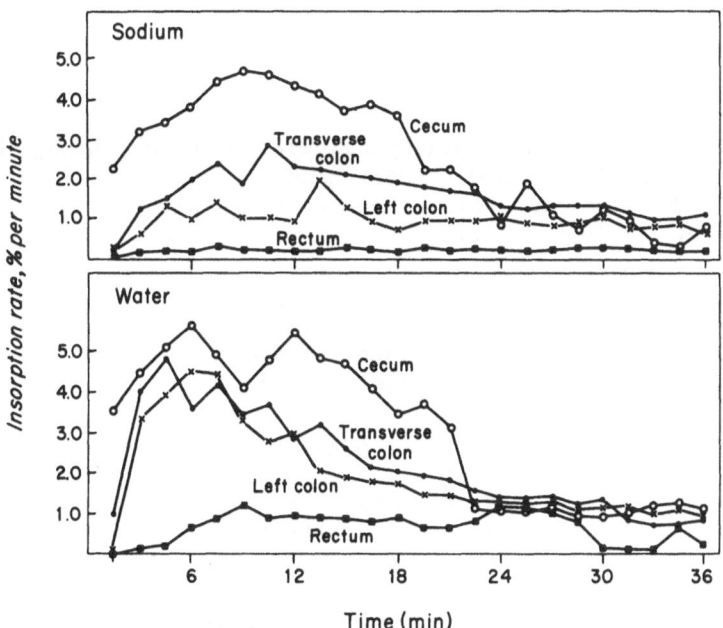

Fig. 3. Insorption rates from the large intestine--effect of time
in one person at each site (from Devroede, et al., 1971).

TABLE 2. Other Materials Absorbed from the Colon

Substance	Quantification (in man)	Comments
Oleic Acid	0.3 - 0.4 g/hr	Colon perfusion
Ricinoleic Acid	0.3 - 0.4 g/hr	Colon perfusion
Octanoic Acid	0.6 g/hr	Colon perfusion
Glucose	?	Passive abs. only
Short Chain F.A.	?	Fermentative products
Amino Acids	?	Passive abs. only
Bile Acids	Appreciable for unconj. B.A.	Passive abs. only

3. Factors that Modify Membrane Function. We know that hormones can modify mucosal function (Phillips, 1969). Levitan showed that mineral-ocorticoids increase sodium and water absorption and decrease potassium absorption. Simultaneously, there is an augmentation of the mucosal potential difference. Levitan also showed that antidiuretic hormone reduces fluid absorption in the colon (Levitan, et al., 1962). Perhaps we should conceive of the colon in terms of its electrolyte conserving function, as akin to the distal renal tubule. It can absorb sodium actively, indeed more efficiently than any other part of the gut, and this active mechanism appears to be under close biological control.

Luminal factors also modify colonic function. Among these are dihydroxy bile acids and C^{18} fatty acids which decrease sodium, water and chloride absorption. These agents also can provoke net excretion of sodium, chloride and water. Figure 4 shows that dihydroxy, but not trihydroxy, bile acids stimulate colonic secretion of water. Ricinoleic acid, the active principle of castor oil, completely inhibits water absorption from the colon. Hydroxy-stearic acid, a bacterial byproduct of oleic acid, has a similar effect, as does oleic acid (Binder, 1973).

4. Chemical Factors that Modify Absorption. Table 3 lists some of the known chemical alterations of fecal substrate. The first three, creatinine, urea and uric acid, will remind you that the colon can be an excretory organ. It is estimated that 20 percent of the total body excretion of urea, creatinine and uric acid occurs via the gastrointestinal tract. Other chemical alterations of substrate have been mentioned earlier; for instance, 7-alpha-dehydroxylation of bile acids, hydration of oleic acid to a hydroxy fatty acid, fermentation of carbohydrates and amino acids to short-chain fatty

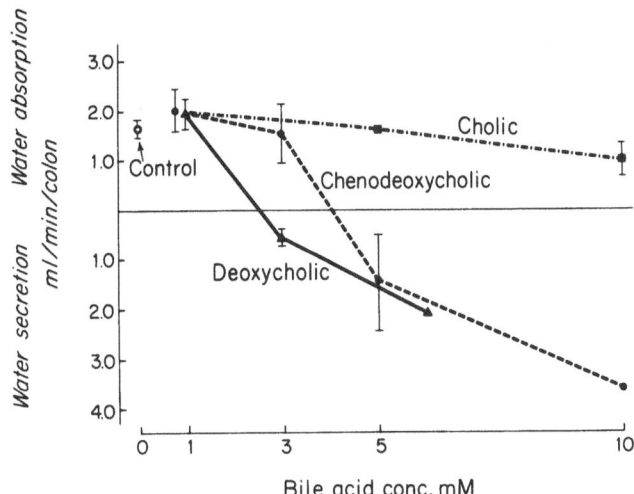

Fig. 4. Effect of different concentrations of deoxycholic, chenodeoxycholic and cholic acid on absorption of water from the human colon (from Mekhjian, et al., 1971).

acids. Carbohydrate fermentation also gives rise to the production of hydrogen. Levitt has used the breath excretion of hydrogen to examine the interaction between substrate and colonic bacteria.

5. <u>Physical Factors that Modify Absorption</u>. Finally, there are some physical factors that modify colonic absorption. We must consider muscular contractility and the transit time of contents as they might modify contact time between the absorbing surface and the contents. Furthermore, we must not forget the heterogeneity of the fecal contents, since they relate to mixing and streaming. Although probably of great importance, these events are difficult to measure <u>in vivo</u>, and the amount of information available unfortunately is very small. Transit time has been measured in relation to absorption during colonic perfusion, but these circumstances are artificial and difficult to relate to circumstances <u>in vivo</u>. Devroede perfused the colon at various rates and showed that with faster rates of perfusion, the volume in the colon increased to a maximum, then reached a plateau (Devroede & Phillips, 1973). Similar relationships also obtained for water and sodium absorption. It is known also that the serum concentrations of drugs vary greatly according to whether a standard dose is given by mouth, by enema into a clean colon, by enema without prior cleansing or by suppository.

In summary, we have some knowledge as to how the colonic mucosa functions, but not much information on the way the colon works in its normal situation; that is, when it is filled with bowel content and feces.

TABLE 3.   Chemical Alterations of Colonic Content

Substrate		Product		Possible Consequence
Urea	--->	Ammonia	--->	
Creatinine	--->	Various N-metab	--->	20% body excretion
Uric Acid	--->	?	--->	
Chenodeoxycholate	--->	Lithocholate	--->	Excretion (? reabsorption)
Cholate	--->	Deoxycholate	--->	Cathartic (? reabsorption)
Oleic Acid	--->	Hydroxy stearic acid	--->	Cathartic
Carbohydrates ? Amino Acids	--->	Poorly absorbed Organic anions	--->	Cathartic

REFERENCES

Binder, H. J., 1973, Fecal fatty acids--Medication of diarrhea, Gastroenterology 65:847.

Devroede, G. J., and Phillips, S. F., 1969, Conservation of sodium, chloride and water by the human colon, Gastroenterology 56:101-109.

Devroede, G. J., Phillips, S. F., Code, C. F., and Lind, J. F., 1971, Regional differences in rates of insorption of sodium and water in the human large intestine, Canad. J. Physiolo. Pharmacol., 49:1754-1759.

Levitan, R., Fordtran, J. S., Burrows, B. A., and Ingelfinger, F. J., 1962, Water and salt absorption in the human colon, J. Clin. Invest. 41:1754-1759.

Mekhjian, H. S., Phillips, S. F., and Hofmann, A. F., 1971, Effect of bile acids on water and electrolyte absorption in the human colon, J. Clin. Invest. 50:1569-1577.

Phillips, S. F., 1969, Absorption and secretion by the colon, Gastroenterology, 56:966-971.

Phillips, S. F., and Giller, J., 1973, The contribution of the colon to electrolyte and water conservation in man, J. Lab. Clin. Med. 81:733-746.

DISCUSSION

R. Levitan: I would like to congratulate Dr. Phillips on an excellent review of the subject. First, an addition to the problem discussed by Dr. Levitt: years ago Dr. James Patterson and I prefused the colon in man with short-chain fatty acids and demonstrated that the entire colon does as well as 30 centimeters of ileum or jejunum in a healthy subject. As far as the absorption of these fats is concerned we have some unpublished information on glucose absorption studies after rectal installation. The glucose disappeared from the rectum very quickly and the levels of glucose in the blood rose substantially. There were, however, some flaws with this technic, because we could not exclude bacterial action and therefore could not be sure that absorption was the only mechanism of glucose disappearance. I always believed that carbohydrates, at least hexoses, can be absorbed by the colon.

I also would like to comment on the general problem of the measurement of colonic absorption. What we are really doing is studying the colon under conditions of diarrhea. All our perfusion technics, in fact, induce diarrhea in a colon that has been completely emptied. Consequently, I have always wondered whether all of these studies are relevant to the events under physiological circumstances. Again, our technics are probably not well suited for study of disease states, because people with colonic diseases cannot tolerate such studies. Furthermore, we have no idea how the different dietary measures influence colonic absorption because we have no technics that permit us to adequately sample solid colonic contents after they have traversed the intestinal tract. Since we have no idea about dietary effects upon colonic absorption in general, I do not know how we can consider the effects of fiber upon absorption. We could feed subjects fiber and study their colonic absorption before and after such a diet. Measurements of transit time and pressure in the colon are very important. Again, this information may or may not be relevant to the "true" physiological state. It seems that we shall have to direct our efforts to improved methodology before we can answer some important questions regarding colonic function. The problem is to devise a method of making a meaningful sample of what was eaten in a regular meal. Until such an approach is available, we have to consider the information about colonic absorption with caution.

It seems possible that our present information about colonic
physiology, which was obtained during perfusion studies, applies
to diarrheal states only.

M. D. Levitt: Dr. John Bond and I have studied the fate of
glucose or lactose that is not absorbed in the small bowel and
therefore reaches the colon. We infused either ^{14}C-glucose or
^{14}C-lactose directly into the cecum of normal human subjects by
a long tube, or into the cecum of rats via a chronically-implanted
cannula. Bond found that when doses of 12.5 g of sugar were infused
directly into the cecum, the $^{14}CO_2$ excreted rose when either the
glucose or the lactose was ingested. There are several possible
explanations for this rapid conversion of intracolonic carbohydrate
to CO_2. When glucose or lactose was infused into the cecum of germ-
free rats, practically no $^{14}CO_2$ was excreted. Thus, bacteria were
necessary for conversion of sugar to CO_2. The bacteria could
aerobically metabolize the sugar to CO_2, or the carbohydrates could
be fermented by bacteria in the colon. The resultant short-chain
fatty acids then could be absorbed by the colon and the actual
oxidation to CO_2 would occur within the body of the rat or human
subject. We investigated this problem indirectly by determining
the maximum amount of oxygen that could be delivered to the lumen
via the blood flow. The amount of oxygen that can conceivably
enter the colon is only about 1/10 to 1/20 of that required for the
observed oxidation of carbohydrates instilled into the colon. Thus

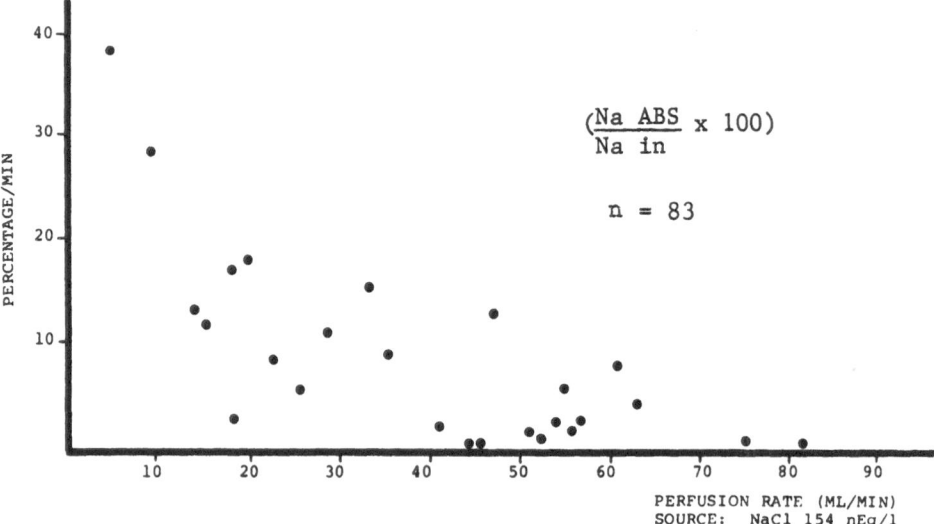

Fig. 1. Sodium ratio absorbed from perfused human colon.

we postulate that the carbohydrates are being fermented in the colon; the short-chain fatty acids then are absorbed and oxidized by the cells of the host. In support of this hypothesis, we found that a variety of short-chain fatty acids instilled into the cecum of germ-free rats were rapidly converted to CO_2. There is a limit to this colonic conservation of carbohydrate, and above about 20 g of carbohydrate, the capacity of the bacteria to metabolize the carbohydrate and the diarrhea is overwhelmed.

   G. J. Devroede: There are three ways to examine the relationship between transit in the colon and absorption. One way is to study patients who do not have a normal transit time. For instance, during colonic perfusions, the times of maximal dye concentration, mean transit time, and total transit time are longer in patients with constipation. If the fluids remain longer in the colon, they will be more completely absorbed. Dividing the proportion of infused fluids absorbed by the mean transit time corrects for this relationship. In the presence of constipation there is a slightly greater absorption, but in terms of proportionate absorption, these individuals do not absorb more than is absorbed by the controls but perhaps slightly less. A second way to examine the relationship between transit time and absorption is to perfuse subjects at varying rates of perfusion. The percentage of the infusate that

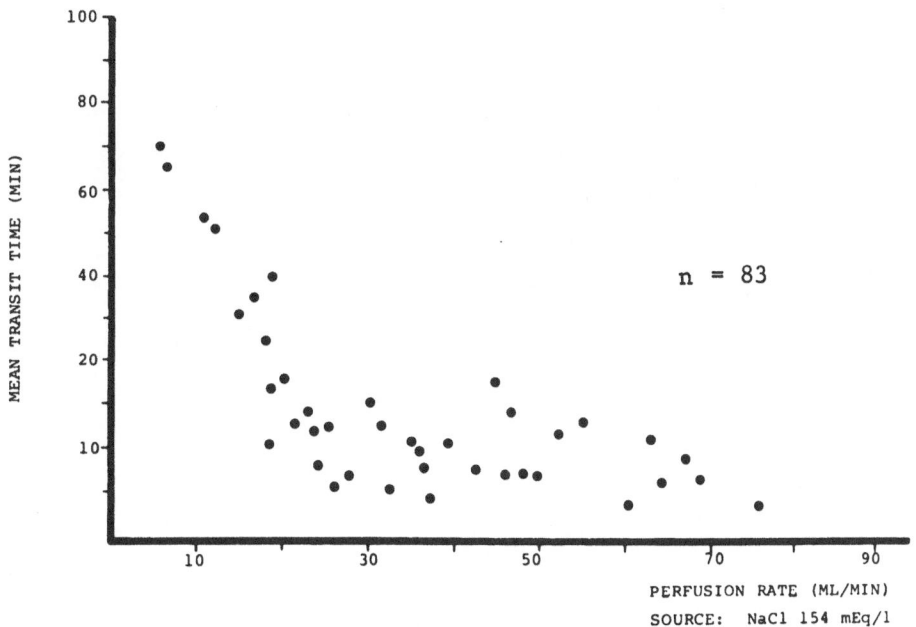

Fig. 2. Mean transit time through perfused human colon.

is absorped decreased with increasing rates of perfusion.
(Figure 1) This is directly related to transit time which decreases markedly with increasing rates of perfusion, the minimum
being reached around 30 to 35 ml per minute. However, as
Dr. Phillips and Dr. Levitan have indicated, these studies are
grossly unphysiological. (Figure 2)

A third way of looking at transit time and absorption is
that of Hinton and Leonard-Jones (1969). Segments of radio-opaque
Levine tube are cut to standard size and are swallowed by the
subject. (Figure 3) The progression of those markers can be
followed and located according to bony landmarks in the right or
left colon, or in the rectosigmoid area. With this method, it was
possible to demonstrate that resection of the nervi erigentes in
a patient resulted in paralysis of the hind gut. In patients with
idiopathic constipation, the transit of the radio-opaque markers
is much slower than normal, and these are quantifiable data. I
know of no study correlating transit and distribution of the
radio-opaque markers with stool weight, frequency, and consistency.
A final point about the relationship between transit and absorption,
is the relationship between motility and potential difference,
which is clearly demonstrated in perfusion studies. (Figure 4)

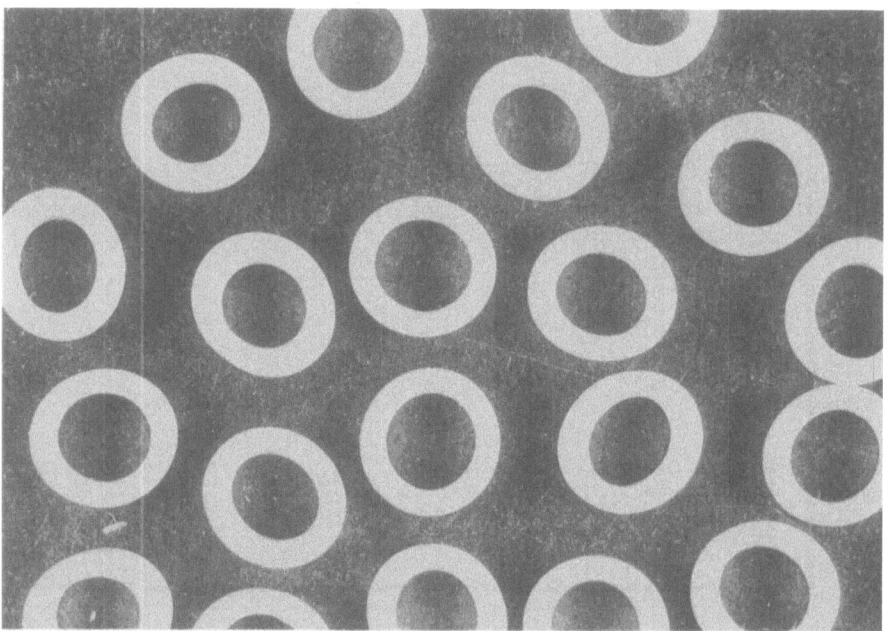

Fig. 3. Segments of radio-opaque levine tube are cut to standard
size.

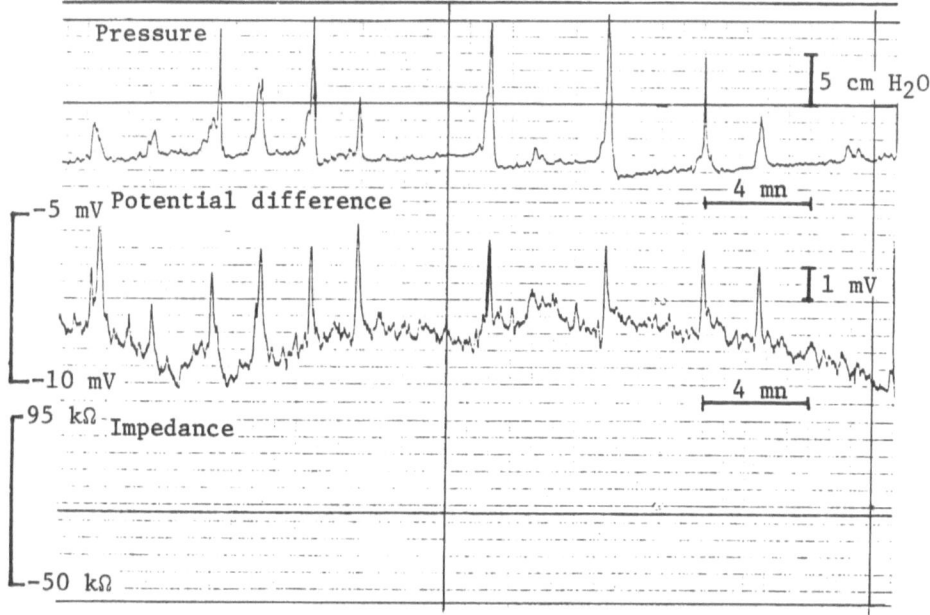

Fig. 4. Relationship between motility and potential difference, which are clearly demonstrated in perfusion studies.

REFERENCE

Hinton, J. M., Leonard-Jones, J. E., and Young, A. C., 1969, A new method for studying gut transit times with radio-opaque markers, Gut, 10:842-847.

ELECTROMYOGRAM OF THE CAT COLON AND COLONIC FLOW

J. Christensen

Department of Internal Medicine, University Hospital

Iowa City, Iowa

The electromyogram of the cat colon is not a subject I planned
to study initially but rather an area that developed as a result
of a casual observation about five years ago. I will summarize in
this paper the work done since then by a group of people who have
collaborated in my laboratory, Caprilli (Christensen, et al.,
1969), Wienbeck, Anuras (Christensen, et al., 1974), Hauser
(Christensen & Hauser, 1971a, 1971b; Christensen, et al., 1972),
and Freeman (Christensen & Freeman, 1972). All of this work has
been published and I apologize for not having anything new and
unpublished to present today.

The electromyogram of the gut has been studied for a long
time. It is well known that in some parts of the gut, that is, in
the distal stomach, small bowel, and colon, the muscular walls
generate signals of two types, slow waves and spike-bursts. The
slow electrical transients, or slow waves, also have been called
pacesetter potentials, electrical control activity and the basic
electrical rhythm. These are slow electrical signals recurring
constantly over time and at very regular intervals. They are not
directly related to contractions. Rapid electrical transients
called spike-bursts occur in such tissues, always occurring in a
small cluster on top of the slow wave. These spike-bursts are
the electrical correlates of contractions. A spike-burst signals
initiation of the contraction but the slow wave by itself does not.
The spike-burst is always phase-locked to slow waves. In the colon,
slow waves differ from those in the rest of the gut in that they
are generated by the circular muscle. The same relationship
between slow waves, spike-bursts and contractions exists in the
colon as in the small bowel. There is a 1:1:1 correlation of

these three events when all three are present. Thus, slow waves
drive the spike-bursts and the spike-bursts are associated with
contractions.

OBSERVATIONS

In studying the colon we have used a preparation of the whole
colon. The entire colon of the cat is removed and everted. A
strip of mucosa is removed from its whole length. The colon is
then mounted on a mandrel and submerged in Krebs solution. Sixteen
electrodes are aligned along its length, spaced at such intervals
that the whole colon is encompassed by all 16 electrodes. We then
can record slow waves from the circular muscle layer from each of
these electrodes separately against a common reference electrode.

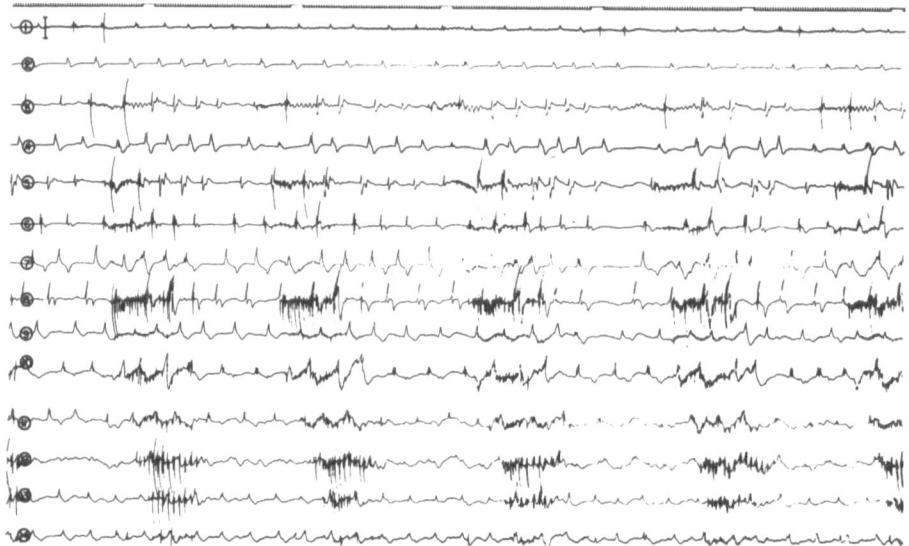

Fig. 1. A record from 14 electrodes equally-spaced along the whole
cat colon in vitro. Each of the 14 tracings represents the mono-
polar record from a single electrode. These are numbered, the
first electrode being the most proximal, adjacent to the ileocecal
papilla and the fourteenth, the most distal, on the rectosigmoid
junction. Time, at the top, is indicated in seconds (ticks) and
minutes (spaces). Slow waves can be seen throughout, accompanied
in some places by bursts of spikes. A pause in the slow waves in
the proximal half of the colon reveals the direction of slow wave
migration. A prolonged complex of intense spike activity can be
seen to move caudad across the distal electrodes at quite regular
intervals (from Christensen, et al., 1974).

The polygraph record thus has 16 channels. Figure 1 shows the
kind of record that is obtained from such a preparation. The slow
waves carry small spike-bursts, most clearly seen in this record
at the proximal end. We can assume that the muscle in this case
is manifesting a brief phasic contraction with each of those slow
waves. Notice that the slow wave is not very regular in the colon.
There is a pause in the slow waves at one point in this record, a
kind of diastolic pause, which reveals the pattern of migration of
the slow waves. They are spreading from about the middle of the
colon backward because that is the direction of phase-lag of the
pause. The other observation in this record is another kind of
signal, a prolonged spike-burst. We have called this the migrating
spike complex. It is a prolonged burst of spikes or, rather,
groups of spikes, which begin in the region of the hepatic flexure
and migrate downstream at quite regular intervals, at a slow
velocity. This migrating spike-burst is seen in all colons studied
in this way. These electrical phenomena also occur in the colon
in situ, as revealed by records from chronically implanted
electrodes in the cat. We know nothing about the controls of
these migrating spike-complexes: we do not know what turns them
on or what turns them off or how consistently they occur in the
colon in situ. They occur always in the colon in isolation.

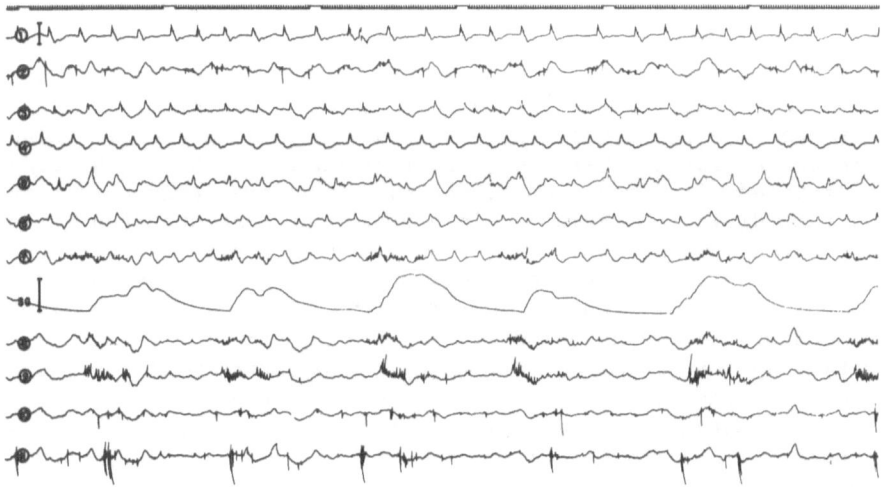

Fig. 2. A record like that in Figure 1, except for the fact that
one electrode has been replaced by a strain-gauge. The strain-
gauge is oriented so as to record contractions of the circular
muscle layer. A prolonged contraction is demonstrated with each
of the prolonged migrating spike complexes (from Christensen,
et al., 1974).

Figure 2 demonstrates that the migrating spike-complex paces
a contraction of the colon, not a twitch or a phasic contraction
but a longer tonic contraction. We simply removed one electrode
and substituted for it a strain gauge sewn to the outside of the
colon so as to record tension in the circular muscle layer. You
see that each time the migrating spike-complex occurred, the
strain gauge registered a contraction of the circular muscle layer.
So the migrating spike-complexes also signal contractions. The
direction of migration of this complex is ahead or downstream
about 70% of the time. The velocity is slow, about 4 or 5 mm
per second. The period of its recurrence is something over a
minute, 77 seconds, and the duration is about 35 seconds on the
average. Thus, three electrical events occur in the colon: slow
waves, phasic spike-bursts associated with slow waves, and migrating
spike-complexes.

SLOW WAVES

I will now discuss the slow waves further. We set out to
examine the gradient of intrinsic slow wave frequency all along the
colon. The reason for being interested in the intrinsic frequencies of the slow waves along the colon is that the direction
of slow wave migration is retrograde, as shown previously, in the
right colon. That direction of migration would predict that if we
examined the intrinsic frequencies they should be lower proximally
than they are distally. After an hour's recording of slow waves,
the 16 electrodes were removed from the colon, and the colon was
divided into rings by cutting between each electrode. The
electrodes were reapplied in their former positions and recording
was continued for another hour. In this way, we divided the colon
into isolated rings and counted the slow wave frequency before and
after that division. Figure 3 is a record of what occurred. Slow
waves in the most proximal region declined in frequency, as they
did at the next two or three electrode sites. In the distal colon,
slow wave frequency actually increased slightly. The other effect
of this division of the colon was to abolish completely the
migrating spike-complexes. Migrating spike-bursts were never seen
in these isolated rings of muscle, suggesting that this phenomenon
requires an integrative mechanism that extends over some distance.
This observation provides an explanation for the normal retrograde
pattern of migration of the slow wave in the proximal colon. Retrograde movement of the slow wave in the proximal colon means that
the slow wave pacemakers in the middle of the colon are so much
faster than those in the proximal colon that the distal slow wave
generators capture the more proximal waves and drive them at a
frequency higher than their native frequency. There is, however,
a phase lag, so that the slow wave appears to spread in that
direction. Beyond the midpoint of the colon the oscillators have

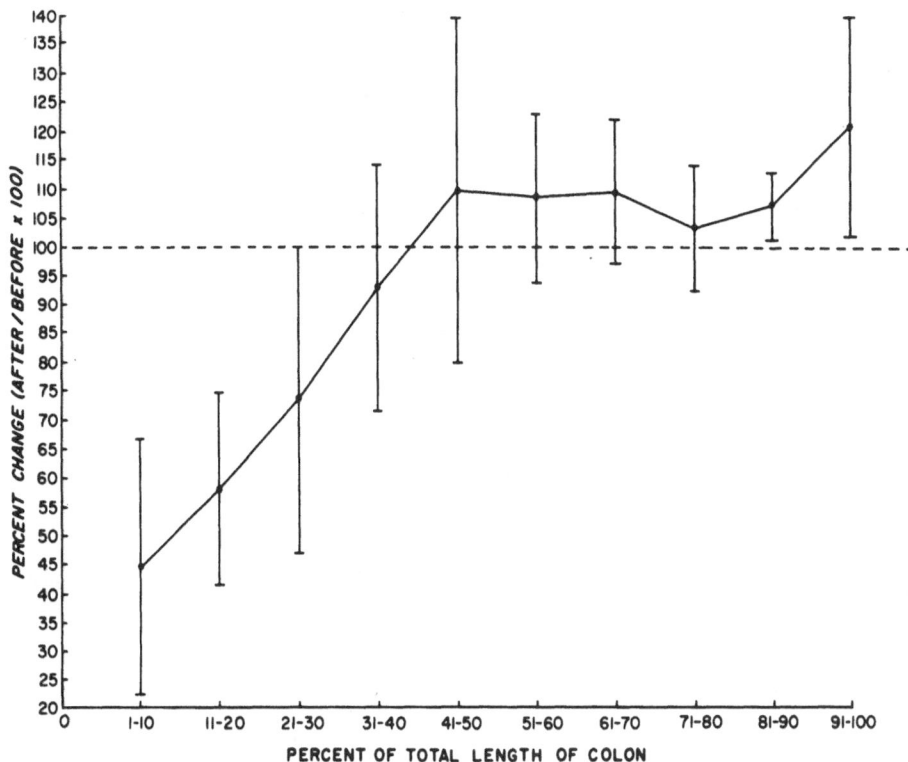

Fig. 3. A graph of the changes in frequencies of slow waves all along the colon produced by its division into rings. The horizontal axis indicates distance along the colon in percentiles, the proximal end being at the left. These are measured from the ileocecal papilla. The vertical axis indicates slow wave frequency in percent change from controls.

the same frequency after they have been isolated (the intrinsic frequency) as they had before. What this means is, that through the middle part of the colon, the slow wave generators probably are working independently and the slow waves never spread very far in either direction. These oscillators are essentially firing independently of each other almost at the same frequency.

The next figure (Figure 4) shows how these two electrical phenomena may be considered. The electrical slow wave is organized in such a way that it seems to begin at a pacemaker which is in the region of the hepatic flexure. It spreads towards the cecum because of the gradient in the intrinsic frequencies of the slow wave oscillators. Throughout the rest of the colon, the slow waves do not migrate very far in either direction. The phasic contractions

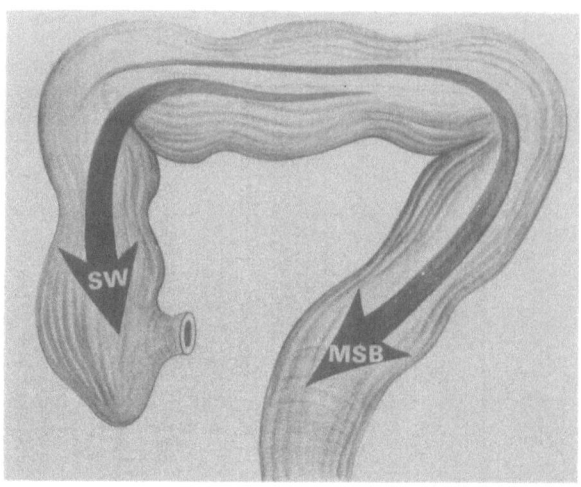

Fig. 4. A diagram indicating the predominant patterns of migration
of slow waves (SW) and migrating spike-bursts (MSB) or complexes
(from Christensen, et al., 1974).

that can follow slow waves would have little effect on net transit
in the middle of the colon, but in the proximal colon those brief
contractions which are paced by the slow waves would have to follow
the slow wave and should produce flow towards the cecum. The
migrating spike-complex, on the other hand, usually begins about
the hepatic flexure and moves caudad. It produces a strong tonic
contraction and it should produce flow in that direction.

There is evidence to suggest that such flow patterns do occur.
In 1904, Elliott and Barclay-Smith examined flow in the colon of
the cat and reported that flow within the colon in situ does what
might be predicted from these characteristics of the electromyogram.
They introduced a thick solution into the exposed colon of the cat.
In the proximal colon, waves of antiperistalsis swept this solution
down into the cecum where it remained for long periods. When they
introduced the solution into the middle of the colon, it was swept
slowly caudad. They described the colon, in fact, as having two
regions. In the proximal region, flow normally was orad. In the
second region, downstream, flow was caudad. They observed this
division not only in the cat, but also in the ferret and other
species.

PACEMAKERS OF THE PROXIMAL COLON

I will now describe other experiments examining the most proximal region of the colon in more detail. In these studies we aligned electrodes along the long axis of the colon in preparations in which it had been opened and pinned flat. The six or eight electrodes all lay within about 4 centimeters of the ileocecal junction and were spaced at intervals of about 1/2 centimeter. The slow waves occurred with a phase lag such that they appeared to arise at a pacemaker beyond the most distal electrode. In the normal cat, a single pacemaker appeared to dominate this segment of the colon about 70% of the time, but it was evident that for the rest of the time more than one pacemaker was operating. Sometimes we could see two, occasionally three, and so on, but as time went on, up to six pacemakers, the maximal number that was permitted by the resolution of the technic, were seen. The predominant state appears to be a condition in which this whole segment is dominated by a single pacemaker. We called that state the coupled or the congruent state. Multiple pacemakers represent varying degrees of incongruence or varying degrees of uncoupling of slow waves in this segment. In the coupled state, when one pacemaker was dominating, it was located within the field of the electrodes for about 80% of the time. For 10% of the time, the pacemaker moved out of the field toward the mid-colon, and the slow waves spread in the reverse direction, i.e., orad through this region. For 3% of the time the pacemaker jumped to the cecal end to produce a pattern of spread such that the slow wave appeared to be arising at the most proximal region. The pacemaker position thus is not fixed; it can move around, presumably because the intrinsic frequencies of slow waves in the proximal colon are not constant. In the small bowel they are quite constant, but in the colon they are not, at least not in the proximal colon. It is my belief that this is the mechanism by which this region of the colon empties itself. If the slow wave pacemaker always were at the hepatic flexure, then the contractions would allow nothing to leave the cecal region. This variability must be a part of the control system allowing the region to be emptied. The migrating spike-complex does not occur in this region and so it cannot be invoked to explain emptying of the proximal colon.

These experiments with the open colon were performed in the summertime and some of the cats came to us with a viral diarrhea typical of cats in animal houses during the summer. It was evident to us from the first that, in diarretic animals, the slow waves were different from those in the healthy animals who had solid stools in the colon. We separated those records from diarretic cats and examined them later. We found that the proportion of time that a single pacemaker dominated the region was different in the diarrhetic animals from that in the healthy animals. In the

healthy cats a single pacemaker dominated the proximal colon for
67% of the time. In the cats with spontaneous diarrhea, the
corresponding figure was 22% of the time. That is to say, more
than one pacemaker could be perceived most of the time in the cats
with diarrhea. We then attempted to produce diarrhea in cats by
giving them castor oil. We gave a small dose the night before the
study and another dose the next morning and assured ourselves that
a liquid stool had been delivered. We then removed the colon,
opened it and studied it. In the castor oil-treated cats, the
figure for the dominance of one pacemaker in this region was 25%,
not significantly different from the 22% figure derived from cats
with infectious diarrhea. On the other hand, cats treated
identically with equal volumes of corn oil did not develop
diarrhea, and dominance of a single pacemaker was found for 72%
of the time in those animals. This observation suggested that the
emergence of more than one pacemaker in this part of the colon is
correlated with the occurrence of diarrhea, whether infective or
induced by castor oil. Slow wave frequencies in the proximal colon
in both the healthy animals and in those treated with corn oil
were about 3 cycles per minute. In the animals with diarrhea,
however, whether spontaneous or castor oil-induced, the frequency
was reduced, as one would predict from a reduction in strength in
slow wave coupling.

We then set out to determine if the effect of castor oil was
direct or not. In this case, healthy colons were mounted and
prepared as I have described for recording from the most proximal
part of the colon. The laxative principle of castor oil, hydroxy-
oleic acid or ricinoleic acid, was added to the bath in the form of
sodium soap at increasing concentrations. We examined the percent
of time that a single pacemaker dominated in this region. With
increasing concentrations of sodium ricinoleate, this figure
diminished from the control value of 67%, and it was significant at
a concnetration of $5 \times 10-7$ M sodium ricinoleate. In another
experiment, the colon was examined for an hour while we recorded
the slow waves and looked at percent of time with congruence: the
sodium ricinoleate was then added so that we had an internal control,
and could thus compare the congruence in the treatment period with
the control hour in each colon. Colons were studied not only with
sodium ricinoleate but also with sodium oleate. The sodium
ricinoleate again produced a dose-related change in congruence.
That is, it induced a dose-related effect, the emergence of more
than one pacemaker for slow waves in the proximal 4 cm of colon,
whereas sodium oleate had no effect. (Figure 5)

We conclude then that the cat colon, which is non-taeniated
colon, generates slow waves in the circular muscle layer very much
like those of small bowel and stomach, and these slow waves pace
phasic contractions. By analogy with small bowel and stomach, the

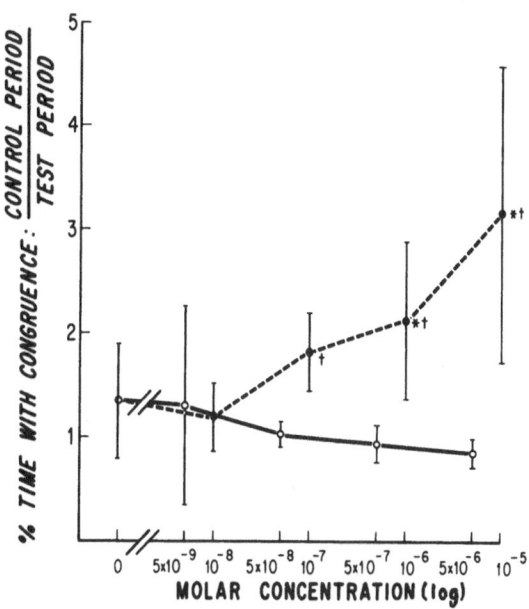

Fig. 5. The effect of sodium ricinoleate and sodium oleate upon
congruence of slow waves in the proximal 3 cm of the colon in vitro.
The horizontal axis indicates the concentrations. The vertical
axis indicates the ratio of the time with congruence (dominance of
a single pacemaker) in the control period to that in the treatment
period. The solid line represents sodium oleate. The dashed line
represents sodium ricinoleate. Asterisks indicate ratios different
(p<0.05) from the average of the controls. Daggers indicate ratios
for sodium ricinoleate different (p<0.05) from those for oleate at
similar concentrations (from Christensen & Freeman, 1972).

direction of spread of these slow waves should be of great
importance on indicating the direction in which the slow waves
pass for most of the time. This pattern of coupling of the slow
wave, so that the phase lag moves orad, is not fixed. Coupling
can be affected by the hydroxy fatty acid, ricinoleic acid but it
is not influenced by oleic acid. Therefore, this uncoupling in
some way most be related to the hydroxylation of that fatty acid.
A similar effect is produced by two other diarrheal agents, quinine
and quinidine, in similar preparations of the cat colon in isolation.
The migrating spike-complex is a phenomenon which seems to govern
flow in the rest of the colon. We do not know anything about the
controls of that phenomenon.

REFERENCES

Barker, J. D., Christensen, J., 1973, Some effects of quinine and quinidine on the electromyogram of the colon, Gastroenterology, 65:773, 777.

Christensen, J., Anuras, S., Hauser, R. L., 1974, Migrating spike bursts and electrical slow waves in the cat colon: effect of sectioning, Gastroenterology, 66:240-247.

Christensen, J., Caprilli, R., Lund, G. F., 1969, Electric slow waves in circular muscle of cat colon, Am. J. Physiol., 217:771-776.

Christensen, J., Freeman, B. W., 1972, Circular muscle electromyogram in the cat colon: local effect of sodium ricinoleate, Gastroenterology, 63:1011-1015.

Christensen, J., Hauser, R. L., 1971a, Longitudinal axial coupling of slow waves in the proximal cat colon, Am. J. Physiol., 221:246-250.

Christensen, J., Hauser, R. L., 1971b, Circumferential coupling of slow waves in circular muscle of cat colon, Am. J. Physiol., 221:1033-1037.

Christensen, J., Weisbrodt, N. W., Hauser, R. L., 1972, Electrical slow waves of the proximal colon of the cat in diarrhea, Gastroenterology, 62:1167-1173.

DISCUSSION

M. Schuster: These are important contributions by one of the leading gut electricians in the United States. To recapitulate briefly in order to emphasize a point, the electrical slow waves reported from the gastrointestinal tract by Dr. Christensen and others represent phasic depolarizations of smooth muscles and are myogenic in origin. Slow waves seem to set the stage for spike-activity and it is the spike-activity, not the slow wave, which is associated with muscle contraction. The slow wave seems to regulate the distance, the speed, and the direction of contractions. Whether or not the spike-activity accompanies slow waves is determined by the algebraic sum of excitatory and inhibitory neural and humoral, and perhaps other, stimuli. These controlling influences as well as the effect of diet are unknown at the present time and remain to be clarified.

Dr. Christensen has described two situations in which diarrhea

occurs in cats; one is a spontaneous, infectious type of diarrhea,
and the other is drug-induced diarrhea caused by agents such as
castor oil and quinidine. By inference, it is assumed that the
disarray of slow waves (the disruption of the normal orad spread
of the slow waves in the right colon) is associated with contractions
that have no polarity and that therefore predispose to the caudad
progress of food and of materials. Since, in fact, the contractions
accompany spike-activity rather than slow waves, it would be of
extreme interest to learn the effects of these two conditions on
observed spike-activity and muscle contraction, and if one can get
flow data at the same time, this also would be highly desirable.
I emphasize this point because it has been demonstrated that a
discoordinated type of segmental activity often leads not to
diarrhea, but to constipation and this is what has led Dr. Connell
and other people to use the term the "paradoxical motility" of
constipation and diarrhea, paradoxical because increased motility
is associated with diarrhea. This is because motility is predominantly segmenting or impeding. Therefore it is equally possible
that the pacemakers Dr. Christensen was describing might lead to
segmentation and therefore to constipation. This is one of the
reasons why it becomes vital to do something that is technically
very difficult, and that is to correlate slow waves, spike-activity,
flow, cinefluoroscopic and manometric data. We also need the
correlates for the slow waves, spike potentials, and the migrating
spike complex in the normal state, in constipation and in diarrhea.

     I should like to ask also whether it is possible to separate
the direct effects of the diarrheal agents on electrical activity
of the gut from the effects of an increased load provided to the
gut with its altered electrolytes in the _in situ_ condition.
Perhaps some of the direct observations on isolated colon strips
might provide an answer. There are, however, many different types
of stimuli which might predispose to diarrhea--quinidine for example,
one of the agents that was used, chelates calcium and this raises
the question then of the effect of calcium and the calcium
dependence of slow waves and spike activity. Magnesium sulfate,
another diarrheal agent, may exert its activity by its well known
effect of releasing choleocystokinin in the small bowel intestinal
mucosa.

     A conference such as this should have a particular interest in
knowing whether species differences in activities relate in any way
to the dietary habits of each species. I am assured by veterinarians
that the diet of a dog more closely resembles the diet of the human
than does that of the cat, with the dog eating a substantial amount
of fiber content and the cat not so doing. There are also
differences in anatomy as was indicated, the cat and dog colon
having no taenia, whereas the human colon does possess taenia.
We have demonstrated that in man at least the slow waves seem to

originate in the taenia coli, then spread to logitudinal muscle and
from there to circular muscle; whereas in the cat Dr. Christensen
has shown quite a different situation.

Finally, it is very tempting to postulate that the differences
in electrical activity between the proximal and the distal colon
that Dr. Christensen has so beautifully shown relate in some way to
differences in embryology, in anatomy, innervation and function.
Embryologically, in the human and the dog the proximal colon
derives from the mid-gut, is innervated by nerves that travel along
the superior mesenteric route, and functions primarily to mix and
dehydrate material. The distal colon, by contrast, derives from
the hind-gut; is innervated by nerves that travel along the inferior
mesenteric route and its functions predominantly are storage and
evacuation when that becomes socially convenient. You have pointed
out, Dr. Christensen, that the migrating spike potential seems to
be peristaltic at times or always. This again, is puzzling because
the colon is quite different from the esophagus in its function and
in its composition. The esophagus is a transit tube and its task
is to move material from the mouth to the stomach. It would not
be needed if the mouth were attached to the stomach, and a giraffe
needs a long esophagus because its mouth is so far away from its
stomach. Esophageal function is primarily that of transit, and
peristalsis is ideally suited, then, to move materials from the
mouth to the stomach. Obligatory peristalsis, however, would be
socially disastrous if it occurred in the colon. I would be very
interested in Dr. Christensen's concept of how the migrating spike
peristaltic situation fits in with the normal non-diarrheal state.

J. Christensen: The migrating spike-complex is always peristaltic and it obviously cannot occur all the time. In this isolated
preparation we have taken it away from its control system and it is
"running free". I think that the migrating spike complex represents
the turning on and off of inhibitory nerves in this preparation, at
least that is a hypothesis for which we have some evidence. You
asked whether the ricinoleate caused contractions. We counted the
spike-bursts on slow waves and computed a contraction index. The
ricinoleate did not change that value from the control state. We
never reported that information because it is an artificial situation.
What should really be done is to record contractions manometrically
in the whole animal. You asked about calcium binding by quinidine.
Of course that happens. The fatty acids also might be calcium
binding agents, but the effects occur with such low concentrations
for the fatty acids and for quinidine and quinine that the amount
of calcium bound would be a trivial fraction of the whole, the
concentration of calcium in the bath being about 2.5 mM. Finally,
you asked whether or not animals with different kinds of diets
might have different kinds of control systems in the colon. I do
not think so, because the mouse, which I presume, eats a high

residue diet, has colonic slow waves like those of a cat. They
have been recorded by Jack Woods in Kansas City.

A. M. Connell: The common feature in diarrheal states is a
tube-like colon. Does the tubular colon result from some sort of
circular movement of the electrical activity?

J. Christensen: I have called this phenomenon fibrillation.
It is a term we all know, though it probably is not accurate. These
dominant slow wave oscillators are moving around from here to there.
I would visualize, on a very slow time scale, a kind of movement
in the colon that might appear radiographically to be a random or
disordered movement, like atrial fibrillation.

FIBER, BULK AND COLONIC ACTIVITY

A. M. Connell

Gastric Laboratory, Cincinnati General Hospital

Cincinnati, Ohio

There is only one point definitely known about fiber and colonic activity, namely that fiber produces a rather larger stool. The rest of the information is speculative. Fantus and his colleagues studied various types of bran and noted an increase in stool weight which varied from 50% to nearly 100%. They also showed that some individuals have a decrease in stool weight of between 16 and 40% when they take additional fiber.

This type of study has been repeated at least several times in different circumstances. Dr. Burkitt, for example, had the imaginative idea of comparing African villagers with English school boys, and came to the conclusion that stool weights in persons who have "natural" diets are greater than those of subjects on the somewhat unusual diet of an English public school (Burkitt, 1974). Similarly, transit time has been shown to be decreased in persons on a high-fiber diet.

Studies of our own demonstrate exactly the same result. In this project, healthy volunteers took as their morning cereal either 1 oz of corn flakes or 1 oz of bran. The average stool weight was 110 g/day for subjects on the low-fiber diet and 240 g for those on the high fiber diet. Transit times were measured by the barium pellet technic from mouth to anus and were found to have decreased on average from 93 hours during the "corn flake period" to 44 hours while taking the "bran".

Dr. Eastwood's group at Edinburgh has performed a similar study, and other groups elsewhere in England and in the United States have obtained similar results. In the Edinburgh study

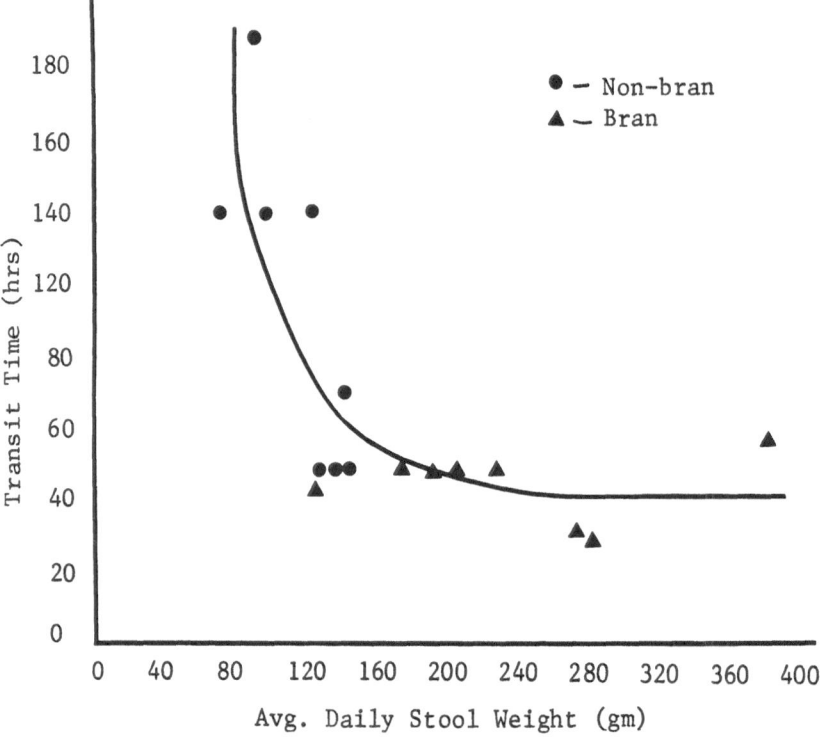

Fig. 1.   Relationship between stool weight and intestinal transit
time in subjects on diets with and without bran.

(Findlay, et al., 1974) the stool weight increased 63% but transit
time decreased less. The plot of the transit time against stool
weight from our own series shows that stool weight seems to be
related to the transit time (Figure 1).   The Edinburgh series
produced a very similar curve, although patients with diverticular
disease were included in addition to normal subjects. Stool
weight may be related exponentially, to the transit time, although
available data are rather scanty to establish this relationship
with mathematical certainty.

    This is all very well. It may be interesting to produce big
stools but does this really prove beneficial? Are we better off
because our stools are bigger, or should we continue along an
evolutionary route of smaller and smaller stools until they disappear
altogether? The relationship of large bulky stools to the intraluminal pressures of the colon is not clear. In the study of
Findlay, et al. (1974) there was a decrease in the overall motility

index in seven patients on a high-fiber diet as compared to a normal diet. These numbers, however, are small.

   If we place a standard bolus in the colon, e.g., a large balloon,
there is a regular increase in the pressure transmitted through the
balloon, as its volume is increased. If volumes are still further
increased, the pressure/volume relationship reaches a plateau. It
is interesting that, in patients with diverticular disease who were
a-symptomatic at the time of study, this phenomenon did not occur.
The diverticular muscle failed to respond to the distending stimulus,
so that increased volume of the balloon did not produce increased
tension in the wall. The question in relation to the diverticular
disease is, if stool bulk is increased, does this help to decrease
the pressures in the colon?

   There are two problems that bedevil all considerations of
this question. One is that the colon is such a variable organ that
studies to date have not really taken account of all possible
factors. Many motility studies have been presented without des-
criptions of the state of filling of the colon at the time of the
study. Most investigators appear to begin with a relatively empty
or clean colon but there is no guarantee that this is always so.
In most studies the patient has been given a somewhat desultory
enema and subsequently tubes are passed into the colon. However,
there may be filling of the colon during the study. I know
personally that from time to time recording tubes become embedded
in the stool during the course of the study and no way to quantitate
this occurrence has been found. Thus, the effect of bulk upon
pressures is seldom noted in pressure studies.

   The second problem is related to the nature of the recording
system itself. In studying pressures, the volume of effective
pressure detectors is of considerable importance, whether the
detector is a small balloon, a large balloon, or an open tube in
a mass of stool or in a segment of empty colon. The following
observations illustrate this problem. In recording intraluminal
pressures from the sigmoid colon using open-ended tubes there is
an exaggerated response to stimuli in persons with diverticular
disease. This exaggeration occurs following stimulation with
morphine and prostigmine (Painter & Truelove, 1964) and with food
(Arfwidsson, 1964). We confirmed that while the motility index
of the sigmoid colon in control subjects doubled after eating,
there was an approximately four-fold increase in patients with
diverticular disease following the same stimulation. However, the
same investigators studying the same general population, but this
time using small balloons, obtained a different result. In this
latter instance, the motility index was doubled in both the control
subjects and the patients with diverticular disease--the apparently
exaggerated response no longer could be elicited.

The explanation lies in a consideration of the relative proportions of the volume of the effective pressure detector and the
diameter of the lumen of the viscus. In the case of a small
volume detector recording from an organ with a relatively wide
lumen there may be many contractions of the wall without any pressure
change being recorded. On the other hand, if the diameter of the
lumen is narrow in relation to the volume of the effective pressure
detector, more alterations in the diameter of the lumen (which of
course reflect motor activity) are likely to affect the pressure-
detecting segment and thus be recorded. Hence the diameter of the
bowel, the nature of the bolus, and its relationship to the effective
pressure-recording segment are important factors in motility
recording, and I do not believe these factors have been adequately
controlled in past studies.

It would be useful to know what happens to colonic motor
activity when a soft pultaceous bolus is introduced into the colon
in the course of pressure studies, but there are virtually no data
on this question. Older studies usually employed a large balloon
which might be considered to represent segmenting activity recorded
from a large bolus, and most illustrations show some motor activity.
However, I do not know that anyone actually has performed the
definitive experiment of recording from an empty colon and then
introducing into it some inert paste to assess the subsequent
effect upon motility.

It could be that in the diverticular situation, where for the
most part the lumen is narrow and the stool consists of small hard
scyballae, a large number of pressure segments, and thus, increased
records of motor activity, are being produced by the nature of the
stool. On the other hand, a bulky, more or less homogeneous
pultaceous stool filling the colon will not have the same pro-
pensity to form pressure segments but will produce a more even
distribution of pressure throughout the colon. It is just possible
that the important factor causing raised intraluminal pressures in
the colon is not a primary and so far undescribed motility defect,
but rather the nature of the stool and the amount of water retained
in it. This in turn would reflect the absorptive and the secretory
functions of the colon.

REFERENCES

Arfwidsson, S., 1964, Pathogenesis of multiple diverticula of the
    sigmoid colon in diverticular disease, Acta Chir. Scand.
    Supplement 342.

Burkitt, D. P., 1974, Dietary fiber and disease, J.A.M.A.,
    229:1068-1074.

Findlay, J. M., Smith, A. N., Mitchell, W. D., Anderson, A. J. B., and Eastwood, M. A., 1974, Effects of unprocessed bran on colon function in normal subjects and in diverticular disease, Lancet, ii:146-149.

Painter, N. S., and Truelove, S. C., 1964, The intraluminal pressure patterns in diverticulosis of the colon, Part II. The effects of morphine, Gut, 5:207-213. Part III. The effect of prostigmine, Gut, 5:365-369.

DISCUSSION

M. M. Schuster: A basic postulate underlying our concepts of the effect of fiber upon colonic motility holds that augmented intraluminal pressures result from underfilling of the colon. For reasons that Dr. Connell has so lucidly presented, bran, because of its effect in increasing stool bulk and weight, is presented as a logical foodstuff to prevent or to treat colonic conditions which are presumed to be associated with some of these increased intraluminal pressures, these conditions being most prominently, irritable bowel syndrome and diverticular disease. Parenthetically, one might add that Dr. Connell has been so successful in "treating" some of his normal subjects with bran that he has increased their stool weight to above the 200 g per day. Fecal numerologists would consider this as diarrhea.

Dr. Eastwood pointed out earlier that water may exist in three phases in relationship to dietary residue. There are: 1) the bulk or free water phase which is independent of dietary residue and is found almost exclusively in diarrhea; 2) the entrapped type of water which is found in the interstices of dietary residue and is marked by PEG; and 3) the gel or non-solvent water which is intimately associated with dietary residue and is inaccessible to PEG. Heaton has described very beautifully the streaming effect which is associated with these various different states of water.

Now, in addition to the streaming effect and the dehydration that results from this, it must be emphasized that the urge to defecate develops predominantly when stool enters the rectum. In those conditions in which the differential in pressure is such that the contents are either impeded from moving into the rectum or actually pressed back into the upper reaches of the descending colon, this call to defecate would not be experienced as often. This would lead to further increase in pressure and to the vicious cycle of even higher progress in an orad direction with the associated orad appearance of the hypertrophic muscles that Morson has described in diverticular disease of the colon.

When normal subjects and patients with diverticular disease
are compared, they are found to differ predominantly in the stimulated state so far as motility is concerned. There does not seem
to be much difference between these two groups in the resting state,
certainly not with the open tip catheters used by Dr. Connell. But
stimulation with morphine, prostigmine, feeding, or with rectal
distension, augments pressures above and beyond those which are
found in normal subjects. Thirty mg of propanthaline can block
these effects.

This raises the question as to the effect of bran upon this
kind of stimulated motility. Is the stimulation simply one of
bulk or are there some biochemical or humoral influences or alterations in flora to account for some of these changes? Would an
extract of bran, for example, have the same beneficial effects as
bran itself? Do other types of fibers, such as cellulose, have
similar beneficial effects? We have heard this morning that there
is some indication that they do not.

There is another interesting aspect of the regulatory features
of bran and perhaps Dr. Heaton could address himself to this
question. An abstract to appear in the 1974 program of the American
Gastroenterological Association is from investigators from Bristol
who have demonstrated that in normal students from private schools
with rapid bowel transit times the transit was slowed by 20 grams
of bran daily whereas in those with slow transit times the transit
was accelerated by bran, and in those with normal bowel transit
times little effect was demonstrated. These observations raise
an interesting question about the "normalizing" nature of materials
of this type.

K. W. Heaton: Dr. Schuster is quite right in saying that we
have gone on record as suggesting that bran normalizes colonic
activity when transit is either unusually fast or unusually slow.
The study in school boys actually was done by Dr. David Payler
(Payler, 1973) and I had the privilege of analyzing the data. He
found, as one would expect, a significant acceleration of slow
transit. There were also in this boys' school population, eating
a typical (low-residue) English diet, five subjects who passed
80% of their pellets in only 23 to 33 hours. In four of these
subjects bran slowed down the transit rate, but because the transit
time in the remaining one was accelerated, the overall change was
not statistically significant. In a separate study that we
published in Lancet (1973, $\underline{i}$, 1278), the time taken to excrete
80% of the pellets was only one day in eight subjects, and when
these individuals were given bran, the transit time of six of them
slowed down to two days.

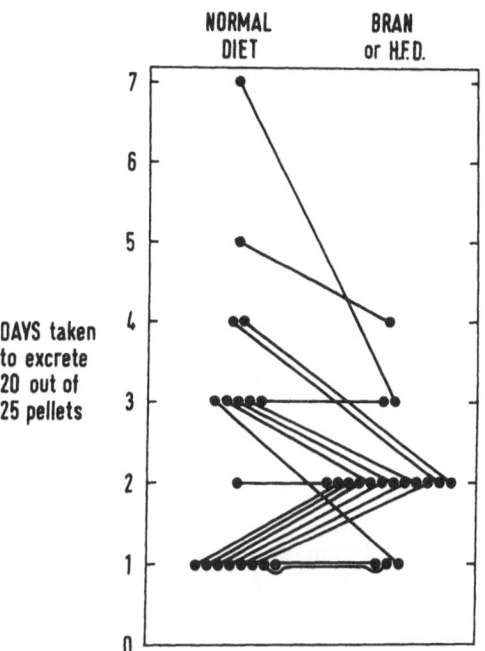

Fig. 1.   Intestinal transit time in 20 subjects before and after increasing dietary fiber intake (from Heaton, et al., 1973).

As Figure 1 shows, the transit times of most of the slow subjects accelerated to two days when they were given bran, and both these changes were statistically significant. We were surprised by this slowing effect of bran but we really should not have been because, as we subsequently discovered, Indians for centuries have been chewing Psyllium seeds, from which we derive Metamucil® and Isogel®, in order to treat both constipation and diarrhea.

M. M. Schuster: I remain puzzled, Dr. Heaton, because, like the Indians who chew Psyllium seed, I prescribe carboxymethyl cellulose as one of the preparations for people who have watery diarrhea, thinking that what I am doing with this hydrophyllic colloid is binding some of that water. This is a different situation from normal school children who are having an increased bowel frequency.

G. J. Devroede: A common mistake pervades the literature in reference to stool weight. Reports usually are made in stool

weights per day and this includes two parameters: the individual
stool weight and the stool frequency. For instance, Winitz, while
studying Vivonex®, demonstrated a marked decrease in stool output
per day in normal subjects (Winitz, et al, 1965). We have done
a similar study with Flexical® which is quite similar to Vivonex:
there was no change in stool weight and a markedly decreased stool
frequency. Another point is that there is a counterpart to
Dr. Christensen's studies in the human colon perfused in situ.
Intraluminal pressure in the right colon becomes very simple, with
only waves of large amplitude and respiratory artefacts. Waves in
the right colon are followed almost instantly by a wave in the
transverse colon, and a wave in the left colon. Output of fluid
at the rectal orifice follows almost immediately.

One point that has never been emphasized is the fact that
during continuous colonic perfusion, output of fluid in the rectum
is not a continuous event: it is discontinuous. For 10 minutes
or so there is no fluid and then 150 or 200 cc of fluid are released; nobody has ever demonstrated where the fluid was retained.
These data would suggest that colonic perfusion possibly measures
events occurring in the right colon where contents are held up by
the pacemaker and that when the right colon is full it contracts
and fluid goes through the left colon. This would explain why
Dr. Levitan did not find any change in electrolyte concentration
between the transverse colon and the rectum. The message we seem
to get from this session is that the right colon and the left colon
are different organs functionally.

A. N. Smith: May I make a comment to strengthen your
conviction that fiber does something to the intracolonic pressures
in patients with diverticular disease. You refer to the small
number of cases. First, these were subjects going through a
fairly complicated sequence of studies with solid and liquid phase
markers, bile acids, and fecal weights.

I hope to show this afternoon that we have kept patients post-
operatively after resection of the colon in diverticular disease
who, as Parks has shown, experience no change in intraluminal
pressures after taking bran for five years. The whole group had
approximately 20 tests and at least 15 of these were after the use
of bran. This is in accord with not only findings on fiber, but
on other bulk-producing agents such as the hydrophilic colloids,
in which Hodgson (1972) has shown similar declines in intraluminal
pressures.

We also have done inadvertently a "control" for the pressure
reduction effect. Someone referred to it earlier, and Eastwood
commented that not all brans are bran. Similarly, some individuals

do not manifest a fall in intraluminal pressure. We have submitted
a paper (Kirwan, et al., in press) which compares nine subjects on
a coarse type of bran which produced a fall in intraluminal pressure,
with another group of nine individuals who were on a floury type
of bran in whom the intracolonic pressures did not fall and the
transit time did not change. The coarse bran was very particulate
and had a high water binding capacity; the fine bran had poor
water-binding effects.

A. M. Connell: Were your studies made on an empty colon or
on a colon that was just as you found it?

A. N. Smith: These were empty colons. I agree with your
comment that we do not know what happens in patients with "natural"
(unclean) colons.

A. M. Connell: If you find changes in an empty colon are you
suggesting that having eaten bran does something to the fundamental
function of the colon? In other words, something has happened to
the physiology of the muscle and it is not just the bulk of
material in the colon that is producing the effect?

A. N. Smith: Both, I think: for instance in the combined
study (Findlay, et al., 1974) we showed that when fecal weight did
not change, the concentrations of both markers fell presumably
reflecting an overfilling of the colon. We have not attempted to
find out if the overfilling affected segmentation. However, I
think that, after a prolonged period of bran treatment, we probably
altered the diameter of the colon. We could only prove this point
if we could show what was happening with feces in situ. This
approach would be much more physiological, but there is a lasting
effect; this should be demonstrated also in the empty colon.

A. M. Connell: The converse can occur in animal models where
diets with very low residue can be used to create the thickened
muscle and a diverticular-like stage.

A. F. Hofmann: When Reiner Polley and I studied patients with
ileal resection, some of whom had bile acid diarrhea and some of
whom had fatty acid diarrhea, we varied the degree of diarrhea by
altering either fat intake or cholestyramine additions to the diet.
Although fecal weight varied over a wide range, if the daily fecal
weight was divided by the fecal frequency to obtain a mean weight
per defecation, it remained very constant in each patient. In
other words, by an analysis of variance, every patient had his own
intrinsic fecal weight which he maintained throughout. When you
increase daily fecal weight with addition of fiber to the diet, does
fecal frequency go up and fecal weight remain constant, or does
weight go up per defecation?

K. W. Heaton: In the schoolboys taking bran, the increase in
fecal weight per day was much greater than the increase in fecal
frequency per day. In other words, the weight of individual stools
increased. In those starting with a slow transit time, mean stool
weight increased from 97 g $\pm$ .42 to .46 SD (p$<$0.025).

None of the schoolboys complained of diarrhea but stool
consistency was not measured in this study. In any case, we do not
know how the preparations of Psyllium seed coat or carboxymethylcellulose act to reduce watery diarrhea.

C. Winans: Do you postulate a mechanism for decreasing the
transit time with increased bulk in those few subjects?

K. W. Heaton: The bulk, or at least the weight of stool was
not increased in the boys who started with a fast transit time,
but only in those who started with slow transit. I have no idea
how the bran slowed the fast transit time.

REFERENCES

Findlay, J. M., Smith, A. N., Mitchell, W. D., Anderson, A. J. B.,
    and Eastwood, M. A., 1974, Effects of unprocessed bran on
    colon function in normal subjects and in diverticular disease,
    Lancet, ii:146-149.

Heaton, K. W., 1973, Lancet, i:1278.

Hodgson, J., 1972, An animal model to study diverticular disease,
    Brit. J. Surg., 59:315.

Payler, D. K., 1973, Food fiber and bowel behavior, Lancet,
    i:1394.

Winitz, M., et al., 1965, Evaluation of chemical diets as nutrition
    for man-in-space, Nature (London) 205:741-743.

PART III

FIBER DEFICIENT DISORDERS OF THE COLON

FIBER DEFICIENCY AND THE IRRITABLE COLON SYNDROME

Thomas P. Almy

Department of Medicine, Dartmouth Medical School

Hanover, New Hampshire

It would be reasonable to question whether a discussion of the irritable colon syndrome should be included in this meeting. The thought is prompted not by any notion that the irritable colon is an unimportant condition, but rather from the difficulties in arriving at a universally acceptable definition of the disorder based upon objective criteria. This uncertainty leads to multiple difficulties in measurement—in being restricted to gross estimates of prevalence at different ages and in different populations, and in accommodating to great uncertainty about its epidemiology and its clinical course. As a result, hypotheses regarding etiology and therapy always have been difficult to validate.

For lack of acceptable data, this discussion cannot be based upon satisfactory empirical observations of prevalence or therapy of the irritable colon. The advice most commonly offered to a patient with this disorder is to restrict the diet to bland and low-residue foods as a means of minimizing alleged stimulation of the bowel. The supposed benefits of this diet have never been separated from the effects of other elements in the total therapeutic program. Neither has a controlled trial of high fiber intakes yet been reported. Therefore, I will attempt to develop a hypothetical basis for a choice of the level of fiber intake from presently available data on the physiology of the colon.

Several groups of investigators (Connell, et al., 1965; Chaudhary & Truelove, 1961; Wangel & Deller, 1965) have supplied acceptable evidence that in most patients with an irritable colon there is increased phasic activity in the distal segments of the bowel. Modest but significant increases over normal in resting

sigmoid activity are found in patients with "spastic colon", and
these differences are exaggerated in the greater response to
stimulation by eating and by neostigmine observed in these
patients. Probably of more importance in determining the state
of excitation of the bowel is the association of sigmoid hyper-
motility with states of emotional tension (Chaudhary & Truelove,
1961; Almy, 1951) considered on clinical grounds (White, et al.,
1939) to be more severe and prolonged than normal in patients with
this disorder. On the other hand, in certain patients with
"functional" diarrhea emotional tension was observed to coincide
with reduction in phasic activity of the sigmoid (Almy, 1951), and
the resting level of motility in these patients is significantly
lower than in other patients with irritable colon, and not greater
than in normal subjects (Chaudhary & Truelove, 1961). Assuming a
relationship between average states of contraction and tension in
the gut wall, we can expect an increase in tension in most but
not all patients with the irritable colon.

     One of the limitations of this reasoning is that our data are
derived, because of the nature of the recording, almost entirely
from the distal colon. If, on the other hand, we measure colonic
motility in terms of the passage time of its contents, we have
evidence from the studies of Manousos and associates (1967) to
indicate that nearly all the patients with irritable colon have a
more active bowel than their normal controls. If we relate this
to Mr. Burkitt's evidence that increased dietary fiber leads to
increased size of stools, and this in turn to decreased passage
time, we have a fundamental basis for agreeing with the concept
that increased fiber would aggravate diarrhea, and for accepting
the clinical impression that at least in this form of the irritable
colon, restriction of fiber would be therapeutically useful.

     But what about the other major form of this disorder--the
spastic colon? What should be the effects of changes in dietary
fiber upon pain and constipation? If the tension in the gut wall
already is increased due to the spontaneous activity of its
muscular coats, should we not experience increased pain if the
bowel is distended from within by a larger fecal mass?

     In experiments involving acute distension of the bowel by an
inlying balloon, Lipkin and Sleisenger (1958) clearly showed that
such distension does give rise to pain, with a pressure threshold
that is an inverse function of the time over which it is applied.
Their studies indicated, nevertheless, that a distending pressure
equal to two to three times the normal pressures spontaneously
generated by muscular contraction can be tolerated for an indefinite
period without pain. It seems unlikely, then, that the gradual
distension of colonic segments attributable to sustained increases
of fecal residues should contribute significantly to the amount of

pain experienced. When Lipkin went further and measured the pressure-volume relationships of the colonic wall during progressive distension from within for 10-15 seconds (Lipkin, et al., 1962), he found a considerable capacity of the wall to accommodate to the distending force. He observed that pain appeared only when the limits of distensibility of the colon were reached and this situation was signalized by a sudden increase in the rate of pressure change. This adaptation, then, is much too fast to be affected by changes in dietary fiber.

Should we not observe a worsening of constipation due to a spastic response of the muscle to distension from within? I submit that the left colon behaves very much like a sphincter, with a relatively high level of resting contraction, and a reduction in its pressure as an essential element in propulsion. This response of the sigmoid is fundamental to Dr. Connell's concept of "paradoxical motility", and was documented earlier by the predictably depressing effect of methylcholine upon sigmoid contractions (Kern, et al., 1949; Davidson, et al., 1955) and by the inverse relation between stool frequency and total sigmoid motility in patients with ulcerative colitis (Kern, et al., 1951). The spasmogenic effect of morphine upon the sigmoid of course is a direct illustration of the relationship of high sigmoid pressures to one form of drug-induced constipation.

What happens to the intraluminal pressure in the sigmoid when the internal diameter (or the radius) is increased by its accommodation to greater bulk of intraluminal contents? Until now we lack a direct answer to this question in patients with the irritable colon, although recent studies on patients with diverticular disease suggest that in them the pressure may be reduced after several months on a high fiber intake (Hodgson, 1972). This finding is entirely compatible with the law of Young and LaPlace, in which

$$T = k\ PR$$

from which I have suggested (Almy, 1965) that

$$P = k\ T/R$$

Unless this principle should prove to be inoperative in the physiological condition of the irritable colon, it seems likely that the propulsion of feces should be aided by increased bulk of the stool.

Thus, in theory I suggest that a high fiber intake should have the following effects upon patients with the irritable colon:

(a) It should aggravate diarrhea, except for those instances in which the term refers only to the frequent passage of small

amounts of mucoid material from the distal bowel when it is
in a state of strong contraction and marked engorgement of its
mucosa.

(b)   It should not increase pain or constipation, and in many
      instances might relieve or decrease both of these symptoms.

I think it important to subject this question of diet in the
irritable colon to empirical trial. So far, uncontrolled trials
are encouraging. The most recent of these shows satisfactory
results for most patients (Piepmeyer, 1974) with relief of pain
and constipation; but the effect on the symptom of diarrhea is not
mentioned. I think the resolution of this question is important
not only because of the high prevalence and the economic significance of the irritable colon itself, but also because of now
acceptable evidence from Scandinavia (Havia & Manner, 1971) that
patients with the irritable colon develop diverticular disease
twice as frequently as matched controls from the general
population.

REFERENCES

Almy, T. P., 1951, Experimental studies on the "irritable colon",
     Am. J. Med., 10:60-67.

Almy, T. P., 1965, Diverticular disease of the colon--the new look,
     Gastroenterology, 49:109-112.

Chaudhary, N. S., Truelove, S. C., 1961, Human colonic motility: a
     comparative study of normal subjects, patients with ulcerative
     colitis, and patients with the irritable colon syndrome.
     I. Resting patterns of motility, Gastroenterology, 40:1-36.

Connell, A. M., Jones, F. A., Rowlands, E. N., 1965, Motility of
     the pelvic colon. IV. Abdominal pain associated with colonic
     hypermotility after meals, Gut, 6:105-112.

Davidson, M., Sleisenger, M. H., Steinberg, H., et al., 1955, Studies
     of distal colonic motility in children III. The pathological
     physiology of congenital megacolon, Gastroenterology,
     29:803-824.

Havia, T., Manner, R., 1971, The irritable colon syndrome, Acta
     Chir. Scandinav., 137:569-572.

Hodgson, J., 1972, Effect of methycellulose on rectal and colonic
     pressures in treatment of diverticular disease, Brit. Med.
     J., 3:729-731.

Kern, F., Abbot, F. K., Almy, T. P., 1949, The action of acetylbeta-
    methylcholine chloride (Mecholyl®) on the human colon, Am. J.
    Med., 7:418.

Kern, F., Almy, T. P., Abbot, F. K., et al., 1951, The motility of
    the distal colon in non-specific ulcerative colitis, Gastro-
    enterology, 19:492-503.

Lipkin, M., Sleisenger, M. H., 1958, Studies of visceral pain:
    measurements of stimulus intensity and duration associated
    with the onset of pain in esophagus, ileum and colon, J.
    Clin. Invest., 37:28-34.

Lipkin, M., Almy, T. P., Bell, B., 1962, Pressure volume character-
    istics of the human colon, J. Clin. Invest., 41:1831-1839.

Manousos, O. N., Truelove, S. C., Lumsden, K., 1967, Transit times
    of food in patients with diverticulosis or irritable colon
    syndrome and normal subjects, Brit. Med. J., 3:760-761.

Piepmeyer, J. L., 1974, Use of unprocessed bran in treatment of
    irritable bowel syndrome, Am. J. Clin. Nutr., 27:105-107.

Wangel, A. G., Deller, D. J., 1965, Intestinal motility in man.
    3. Mechanisms of constipation and diarrhea with particular
    reference to the irritable colon syndrome, Gastroenterology,
    48:69-84.

White, B. V., Cobb, S., Jones, C. M., 1939, Mucous colitis,
    Psychosom. Med. Monographs #1.

DISCUSSION

A. M. Connell: First I want to follow up your very apt comment
about the fact that we are children of our generation. As I
indicated to you this morning, we are studying sophomore medical
students who are a very well-behaved, starry-eyed but somewhat
malnourished group of young men and (a few) women and many of them
are rapturous about the fact that we are doing a study with
"natural" foods. Several points occur to me in relation to this
paper. I think that the irritable colon situation is related in
some way to changes in luminal diameter or the degree of luminal
segmentation. The nature of the colonic content requires the most
serious consideration in interpreting the significance of pressure
studies. Alternatively, the perfusion situation also is artificial
and a "natural" colon is very difficult to study. There is all
the difference in the world between the activity of a colon filled
with small hard marbles of stool and a colon that has a continum

of pultaceous material which presumably acts as one single fluid
phase, albeit a heterogenous one.

    We think that bland or natural fiber helps the irritable colon
situation. I suppose most clinicians who have treated patients
with natural fiber know that they all return initially reporting
they are delighted. But in the irritable colon situation, uncontrolled studies do not really tell us much because the placebo
effect is significant. One hesitates to recommend a controlled
trial in patients with the irritable colon because it is a
difficult situation to define and to control. I do not think any
of us is going to be convinced that fiber helps until decisive
unbiased data have appeared. Dr. Almy hinted that the irritable
colon syndrome is a precursor of diverticular disease. I do not
know whether this is so or not, but much of the information is
highly circumstantial. The motility features of the two conditions
in certain respects are similar, for example the frequency of the
contractions, that is, the amplitude of the response to stimuli.
On the other hand, there is the undoubted fact that many patients
appear in the hospital with severe diverticular disease with a
very brief attendant history. It may be that diverticular disease
is the end result of a number of pathophysiological states. No
doubt many patients with diverticular disease have not had previous
symptomatic irritable colon although clearly the process may have
been developing silently.

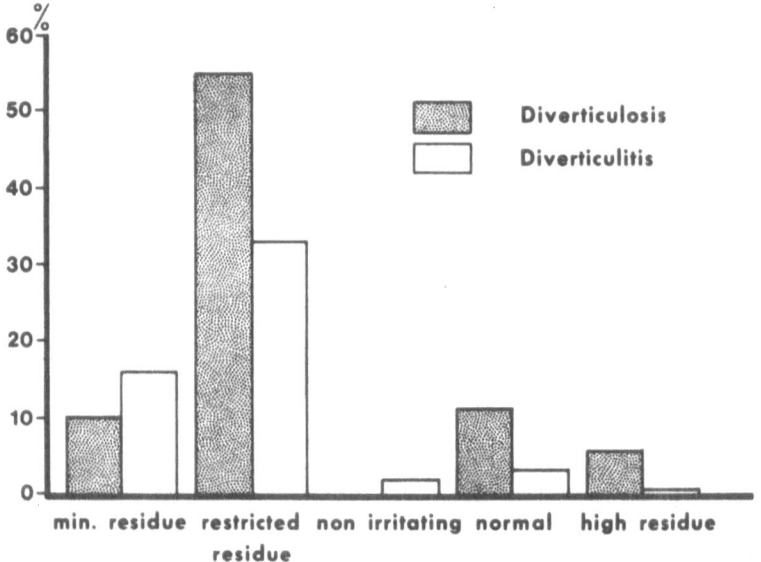

Fig. 1. Types of diets prescribed for patients with diverticulosis
and diverticulitis in hospitals in Canada.

G. J. Devroede: Figure 1 shows what the conflict between orthodox and heretics has created in Canada. You can see what is presently being prescribed in diverticular disease: on the left side are hospitals using minimum-residue diet, and on the right are those using a high-residue diet, with the majority being careful and adhering to the low-residue diet. Another point that has not been discussed today, has to do with Miller's studies. These investigations have shown that the rat is capable of selectively contracting or relaxing the colon in response to "a reward mechanism". This is another factor that we must take into account: not only the content of the bowel, but the container.

H. M. Spiro: The work of Neil Miller involves placing tubes into the open brain at the so-called reward center; the rat's intestine is laid wide open and when the intestine contracts, he stimulates the reward center. It is quite miraculous to watch how the intestine will contract repeatedly. Then, whenever the tightly-contracted intestine relaxes a little, he stimulates the reward center again, and the intestine will open up again. These observations, of course, parallel transcendental-meditation alpha bio-feedback and other current psychologically-influenced approaches. We must recognize, however, that reward for a rat that probably does not think about tomorrow too much is a little different from a reward for human behavior.

DIVERTICULAR DISEASE (PATHOLOGY)

A. B. Price

Department of Pathology, St. Mark's Hospital

London, England

Perhaps Professor Arthur Keith, who described the pathology of diverticula of the alimentary tract in an article in the British Medical Journal in 1910, should be the person to deliver this paper (Keith, 1910). If alive today he would be 110 years old and hence a little elderly for flying the Atlantic! In that paper he described colonic diverticula as true invaginations of the epithelium through the bowel wall, caused probably by increased luminal pressure. He noted that the taeniae were contracted and the circular muscle was thrown into folds, like a concertina. He also observed that diverticula occurred at points of weakness in the colonic wall where it was penetrated by blood vessels. Since that publication, surgical pathologists have been able to improve but little on the description of the pathological changes in diverticular disease.

The sigmoid colon is involved in diverticular disease in about 90% of cases. In most Western communities 10% of people over the age of 40 have evidence of diverticular disease, and over the age of 70, one person in three will show evidence of the disease. It may be a little unjust to belittle the contribution of modern pathologists for they have been responsible for a shift in emphasis away from the diverticulum and to the muscular abnormality. With the clinicians, they have introduced the concept of diverticular disease.

Diverticular disease includes the three conditions listed in Table 1, which also gives the occurrence of these abnormalities in an old St. Mark's Hospital series. The abnormality of colonic muscle is one of the key factors in relating the role of fiber

TABLE 1. Types of Diverticular Disease in a Series of 173 Patients
at St. Mark's Hospital, London, England

Muscle abnormality and diverticulosis + diverticulitis	112 64.7%
Muscle abnormality + diverticulosis	56 32.4%
Muscle abnormality only	5 2.9%

deficiency to the pathogenesis of diverticular disease. As
Painter will point out in the next paper, the sigmoid colon under-
goes intermittent segmentation. This ensures mixing of the fecal
stream. On a low-fiber diet the reduced diameter of the colon
results in the development of high segmental pressures with
consequent pulsion diverticula (Painter, et al., 1975). Before
describing the end results of a life of "low fiber", I should like
to emphasize certain aspects of the normal anatomy of the colon.

The circular muscle forms a continuous band around the colon.
The longitudinal muscle, external to this, is mostly gathered into
three bands. This arrangement divides the colonic wall into two
lateral inter-taenial areas and an anti-mesenteric area. The vasa
recta brevia and vasa recta longa branches of the terminal arcades,
penetrate the bowel wall in the lateral inter-taenial regions. It
is at these points that diverticula are most commonly found: that
is, in two parallel rows in the lateral inter-taenial regions.
These are the points of inherent weakness in the colonic wall that
were stressed by Keith in 1910.

I wish to concentrate here on the colonic muscle abnormality
(Morson, 1963) which can manifest one of several patterns. The
taeniae often are thickened and shortened (Williams, 1965), being
classically described as of cartilaginous consistency. The
circular muscle may be arranged in one of three ways: circular
bands due to localized thickening; circular bands due to simple
infolding; and uniform thickening (Hughes, 1969). In the commonest
form with localized thickening, the bands do not encircle the
whole bowel but form a series of interdigitating semi-lunar arcs,
each band fading out in the region of the mesenteric taenia on one
side and the anti-mesenteric border on the other. This arrangement divides the colonic lumen into a series of segmental chambers.
(Figure 1) It is from these chambers that the abnormal pressures

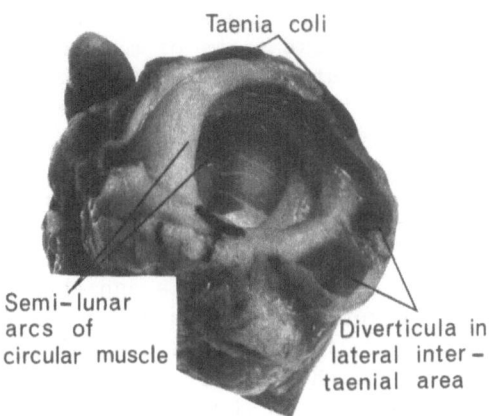

Fig. 1. Abnormal patterns of muscle thickening in diverticular
disease. The bowel is divided into a series of segmental chambers
by the thickened muscular bands with diverticula in each chamber.
(The taenia are indicated in black.)

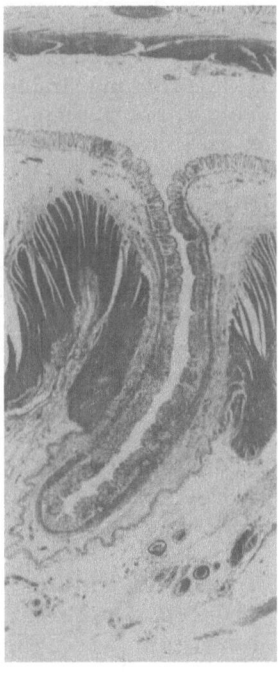

Fig. 2. A sigmoid diverticulum with uniform muscular thickening on
either side. Above is a piece of normal sigmoid colon for comparison.

are recorded. In the uniform type of muscular thickening strictures
may result even when diverticula are absent. Histological examination (Figure 2) confirms these forms of muscle abnormality but
has not yet answered the question of whether the thickening is due
to hypertrophy or hyperplasia of the muscle fibers (Arfwidsson,
1964; Slack, 1966; Williams, 1965).

I already have mentioned that 90% of diverticular disease
affects the sigmoid colon, but other regions can also be involved,
usually those in continuity with the sigmoid. The entire colon
may be involved, showing both diverticula and the muscle abnormality.
In some cases only the right side of the colon is diseased. Right-
sided colonic diverticular disease is of special interest as it is
not usually associated with the muscle abnormality. Furthermore,
it occurs in a younger population than does left-sided disease,
and is the commonest form found in certain non-Caucasian populations.
In a study of a Japanese population in Hawaii with diverticular
disease, 60% had only right-sided involvement.

While most of the pathological findings in diverticular disease
can be explained within the context of the current theory of fiber
deficiency (Painter & Burkitt, 1971) and the subsequent disturbance
in colonic pressures, certain anomalies remain. Diverticular
disease can occur without the muscle abnormality and the muscle
abnormality can occur without diverticular disease (Fleischner,
1971). Right-sided disease occurs and indeed is the commonest form
in certain non-Caucasian groups. A recent Indian study (Antia &
Desai, 1974) has shown that in a population taking a high-fiber
diet, 23% of that population aged over 70 years, exhibited diverticula on barium enema. This suggested that a difference in
longevity might account for much of the difference in the incidence
of diverticular disease between Western and Afro-Asian populations.
Indeed, in the most recent demographic yearbook the life expectancy
of inhabitants of the African continent is given as only 45 years.
A recent study from Greece (Manousos, et al., 1973) compared the
incidence of diverticular disease in urban and rural communities.
Although the incidence was higher in the urban community, the
roughage in the diet of the two societies was considered to be the
same. These authors suggested that the difference might be a
reflection of the sociological tensions in urban living, rather
than a difference in fiber intake.

We have heard Dr. Devroede, in discussion, state that because
two things occur together they do not necessarily cause each other;
and to illustrate this we have heard of spurious correlations
between certain diseases and the sale of ice creams, tin cans, and
even the level of rainfall. This warning should be heeded when
considering diverticular disease and dietary fiber intake.

REFERENCES

Antia, F. P., and Desai, H. G., 1974, Colonic diverticula and
    dietary fiber, Lancet, 1, p. 814.

Arfwidsson, S., 1964, Pathogenesis of multiple diverticula of the
    sigmoid colon in diverticular disease, Acta Chir. Scand.
    (Suppl), 342.

Fleischner, F. G., 1971, Diverticular disease of the colon,
    Gastroenterology, 60:316-324.

Hughes, L. E., 1969, Postmortem survey of diverticular disease of
    the colon, Gut, 10:336-351.

Keith, A., 1910, Diverticula of the alimentary tract of congenital
    or obscure origin, Brit. Med. J., p. 376.

Manousos, O. N. and Vrachliotis, G., et al., 1973, Relation of
    diverticulosis of the colon to environmental factors in
    Greece, Am. J. Dig. Dis., 18:174-176.

Morson, B. C., 1963, The muscle abnormality in diverticular disease
    of the sigmoid colon, Brit. J. Radiol., 36:385-392.

Painter, Neil S. and Burkitt, D. P., 1971, Diverticular disease of
    the colon: a deficiency disease of Western civilization,
    Brit. Med. J., 2:450-454.

Painter, N. S., Truelove, S. C., Ardran, G. M., and Tuckey, M.,
    1965, Segmentation and the localization of intraluminal
    pressures in the human colon, with special reference to the
    pathogenesis of colonic diverticula, Gastroenterology,
    49:169-177.

Parks, T. G., 1968, Postmortem studies on the colon with special
    reference to diverticular disease, Proc. Roy. Soc. Med.,
    61:932-934.

Slack, W. W., 1966, Bowel muscle in diverticular disease, Gut,
    7:668-670.

Williams, I., 1965, The resemblance of diverticular disease of the
    colon to a myostatic contracture, Brit. J. Radiol.,
    38:437-443.

DISCUSSION

H. M. Spiro: I gather that you feel as Connell has suggested,
that there are a large number of patients who have no colonic
muscular abnormalities. Is that right?

A. B. Price: I wouldn't say a large number, but...

H. M. Spiro: Can you give us some idea of how often in the
past six months you actually have seen the muscular abnormality in
a resected specimen? I ask because while my colleagues show me
photographs through the colonoscope of what I take to be the
muscular bands, my colleagues in pathology do not show them to me
very often.

A. B. Price: Unfortunately, I do not have the precise
figures. My impression is that about 10% of specimens do not
have a muscular abnormality in the sigmoid colon. The other
observation that worries me is that the muscle abnormality often
is confined to a short segment of the sigmoid colon. Proximally,
the abnormality often fades out, even though diverticula are
present. An additional difficulty in interpretation is that the
normal sigmoid colon is, in any case, thicker than the rest of the
colon.

A. M. Connell: The real problem in all this is which comes
first? Does this muscle abnormality really exist? Does it cause
high intracolonic pressures? Or do high pressures from the
irritable colon cause muscle abnormalities? Assuming that the
muscle abnormality may occur or that high pressures may develop
because of scanty bulk in the stool, can we go further and say
that if we increase the bulk, we will affect or reverse this
situation? Even our so-called hard stool has considerable resistance to compression but the soft stool accompanying a high-fiber
diet could have little effect, in a mechanical way, on this rigid,
almost cartilage-like muscle.

R. Wissler: I was particularly interested in several points
in Dr. Price's abstract which were not discussed in his paper.
He pointed out that there is a marked difference between the
incidence of muscle abnormality in the surgical and autopsy series
of diverticulosis. This may be due to the fact that the autopsy
pathologist does not take the time to look for such abnormalities
unless he is particularly interested in this disease. I think
that there is a real problem here, in terms of what comes first--
the muscle abnormality or the diverticulosis. I would like to
ask Dr. Price to comment on this discrepancy.

I was also interested in his reference to the recent study of Greek urban and rural communities, in which no significant relationship between fiber intake and diverticulosis was established. I suppose this study is similar to the Indian series previously mentioned. The incidence of diverticulosis may have less to do with fiber deficiency per se than with the total life-style. I was told by the pathologists with whom I trained that diverticulosis was a disease of civilization. Does it correlate with the mores of polite society which require keeping up the pressure in one's colon? What other correlations exist with the requirements of Western civilization?

I think that the treatment of this disease also is enigmatic. I would like to hear the views of Dr. Price and others about its reversibility. Having studied smooth muscle cells for a number of years, I think that, given removal of the stimulus, diverticulosis might be reversible, regardless of whether it is a hyperplasia or hypertrophy. On the basis of my limited knowledge of the treatment of this disease, I believe that the average gastroenterologist--not at the University of Chicago, but perhaps elsewhere-- would probably treat it with a bland, low-residue diet. If the disease is indeed reversible, and if fiber does play an important role, then such a treatment appears unsatisfactory.

H. M. Spiro: Bland diets, low-residue diets, and restricted-fiber diets are all separate items and the idea that one would use a bland low-residue diet is a meaningless term. We talk about the amount of fiber in a diet and not the amount of residue in the diet.

D. P. Burkitt: It is a fallacy that because the average age in Africa or India may be only 45 years, that therefore there are no old people. The average age is around 45 because often 50% of the children die before they reach the age of five. But in South Africa it has been shown that if Africans reach the age of 45 they have a far better chance than Europeans to reach the age of 90. A recent survey in Uganda has shown that about 6% of the population are over the age of 60 which compares with 14% of the population in England over the age of 65. So that although there are fewer old people, there are far more than is generally believed. There are about 2-1/2 times the proportion of people over the age of 50 in the United States as there are in India.

Now, with regard to this recent report from the Lancet (Antia & Desai, 1974). It is a puzzle and is at total variance with all the other figures we have from India. There is a very large university department of radiology in Delhi where the professor has been particularly interested in diverticular disease, and in 16 years he has detected only nine cases. Similar figures are available from Calcutta and from Dacca in Bangladesh. I believe that one of the two hospitals quoted in the Lancet article was for Parsees who consume a more Western type of diet than do the Hindus or the Muslims in India.

A. B. Price: I would like to clarify some points for Dr. Wissler. In my abstract the comparisons of autopsy and surgical series were from the works of Hughes (1969), Parks (1968) and Morson (1963). I suggest that the higher incidence of the muscle abnormality in the surgical series might reflect a change responsible for symptoms, rather than being the prime pathological event. The Greek study that I discussed is the work of Manousos (1973).

FIBER-DEFICIENCY AND DIVERTICULAR DISEASE OF THE COLON

Neil S. Painter

Manor House Hospital

London, England

Diverticular disease of the colon has become a clinical problem only in the last 70 years, the traditional life-span of man. Any clinical student of today would recognize a barium enema showing colonic diverticula but, in 1900, Telling of Leeds in England could not find anyone who knew anything about diverticulitis. Colonic diverticula had been described in 1845 but were regarded only as a pathological curiosity until 1900.

The relationship of diverticula to the segmental arteries that supply the colon is well known, but I would like to emphasize that these arteries only select the commonest site of diverticula. They cannot be held responsible for the mucosal herniation, since the anatomy of the colon is the same in those races and communities which do not develop diverticulosis.

Since diverticula are hernia, they must be ascribed to a weakness of the bowel wall, to abnormally high intracolonic pressures or to a mixture of these two factors. Hence, many theories have been put forward as to the pathogenesis of this disease. Despite a great deal of work, no congenital weakness in the colonic wall has ever been demonstrated. Thus, for practical purposes, it is an acquired disease. Apparatus capable of recording the pattern of the intracolonic pressures accurately and continuously over long periods only became available in the last two decades and it was only then that pressure-recording coupled with intermittent cineradiography revealed that segmentation of the colon was responsible for producing high localized pressures that forced the mucosa through its integument (Painter, 1962 and 1964; Arfwiddson, 1964).

The segments of the sigmoid which bear diverticula produce, on the average, more total pressure, and pressures of a greater amplitude than do segments of the normal sigmoid, or apparently-normal segments of the sigmoid in patients with diverticular disease. This differential capability of the diseased segments is accompanied by local thickening of the colonic muscle. This thickening precedes the actual appearance of diverticula, as does the ability of segments whose muscle is thickened to produce high pressure. This state of affairs corresponds to the "pre-diverticular state" of earlier writers (Painter, 1962 and 1964; Arfwidsson, 1964; Painter and Burkitt, 1971).

The mechanism responsible for the production of high localized intra-sigmoid pressures was demonstrated by placing three open-ended water-filled polythene tubes into the sigmoid, recording pressure continuously and then using cineradiology to correlate the configuration of the colonic wall with the intraluminal pressures. The segmentation mechanism of pressure production is shown diagramatically in Figure 1. Some frames from a cineradiographic film of a man of 45 with diverticulosis were published by Painter and his colleagues (1965) with the pressures recorded from the immediate vicinity of a diverticulum. A wave of pressure which rose to 60mm/Hg caused this diverticulum to be further extruded. The relationship of segmentation to the pathogenesis of diverticula may be illustrated by squeezing mud between the fingers of the clenched hand. The fingers represent ridges of a colonic muscle which compresses the mud which escapes between the fingers. The colonic mucosa is driven between gaps in the circular muscle in an essentially similar fashion.

So much for the mechanism responsible for diverticula. Historically, diverticula were known to be of no clinical consequence until the first ten years of this century. In 1900, diverticulitis did not "exist" but in the next decade its complications surprised even surgeons of repute so that, by 1920, Bland-Sutton likened it to that "new" disease appendicitis and described it as a "newly discovered bane of elders". By 1925, it was so common that its radiographic appearances had been described by Spriggs and Marxer (1925).

GEOGRAPHICAL DISTRIBUTION AND RELATION TO DIET

Looking at the geographical distribution of the disease throughout the world, it is common among white Americans and Europeans. It is common in the American black and in the West Indian who has lived for many years in Britain, but is rarely seen in their forebears in rural Africa, although it is beginning to be reported in Africans who live in large towns and who have adopted Western eating habits. The disease has appeared in Japan only recently, although it is very

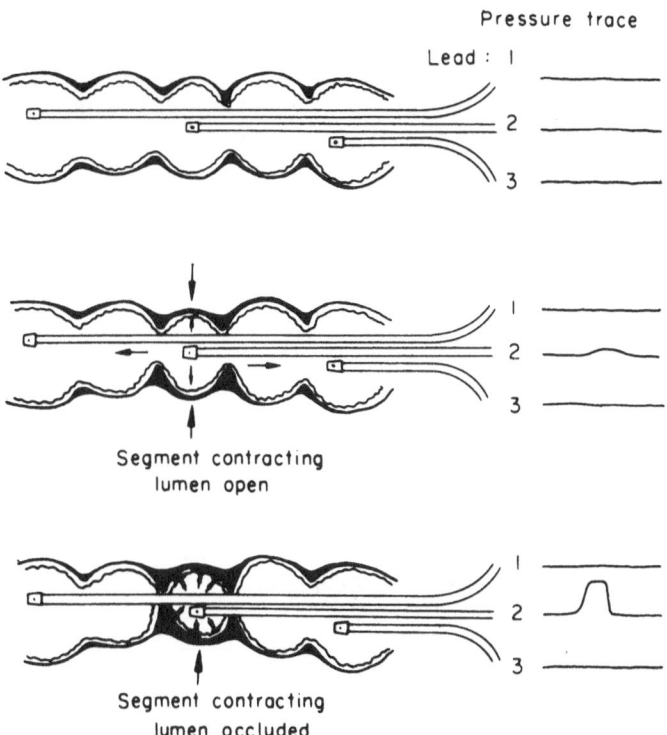

Fig. 1. Diagram to show mechanism of production of localized intra-colonic pressure. This depicts open-ended recording tubes in longitudinal sections of colon, with the pressure tracings that would be derived from them. The <u>top</u> section shows a colon with haustral markings but with its lumen open. Changes of pressure brought about by small movements of its walls would be able to disperse rapidly along its open lumen and so no significant change in pressure would be recorded as no resistance to the movement of the colonic wall would be offered other than that due to the viscosity of its contents. The <u>middle</u> section shows a segment contracting when the lumen on each side of it is narrowed, but not occluded by contraction rings. This segment's contents would be forced through the narrowed bowel on either side and the resistance to their flow thus encountered would result in a rise of pressure being recorded by Lead 2; the other two leads, being in open bowel, would be virtually unaffected. The <u>bottom</u> section shows a segment isolated from its fellows by contraction of the rings that bound it. Obviously, high pressure would be generated in this segment if it contracted; furthermore, this pressure would be localized to this segment and only be recorded by Lead 2 (from Painter, et al., 1965).

common in Hawaiian Japanese who have been reared on an American diet (Painter and Burkitt, 1971).

Hence, the disease is not due to racial differences and must be related to a change in the colon's environment, and this would be affected by that part of our food which is least altered by digestion and so reaches the colon almost unchanged. This is the fiber fraction of our food. In England, fat consumption has increased by about one-half since 1870, sugar consumption has doubled, and, using the millers' own figures, the cereal fiber eaten has decreased to about one-tenth. This is due to the finer flour produced by roller milling and to a decreased consumption of bread and flour products; so this change in fiber consumption has a profound effect on the quantity and the quality of the stools.

The transit times and stool weights in Britain may be as long as five days and the daily amount of stool passed weighs slightly more than 100 g of hard feces (Table 1). English vegetarians, who eat more fiber, pass about 200 g of feces daily with a transit time of less than 50 hours. This corresponds to the figures derived from African students who ate a partly European diet; they passed an average of 185 g daily with a 47-hour transit time. By contrast, rural Ugandans had a transit time of only 35 hours and passed no less than 470 g a day of soft unformed stools without the need to strain. As a result of this observation we gave bran to some patients who were straining and this increased their daily stool weight to about 200 g and reduced their transit time to less than 50 hours. Hence, the fiber content of our diet alters the behavior of the bowel profoundly (Burkitt, Walker and Painter, 1972).

If we consider the role of segmentation as shown diagramatically in Figure 2, it is obvious that the viscosity of the fecal stream will have a profound effect on the pressures required to propel the colon's contents. Soft stools will pass through the bowel with little effort but the colon will have to segment vigorously and produce high pressures if the stools are hard.

I believe that if the colon has to propel hard stools for 40 years as opposed to soft bulky ones, it must overwork to produce abnormally high pressures. Over half a lifetime, the sigmoid hypertrophies; its muscle thickens and is thrown into ridges between which there are gaps. This is the "pre-diverticular state". Finally, the mucosa is driven through the muscular coat by the force of the intracolonic pressure as the colon struggles with an abnormally hard stool. The pathogenesis of colonic and vesical diverticula is thus essentially similar (Painter, 1962, 1964; Painter and Burkitt, 1971).

TABLE 1. Transit Times as Shown by Hinton's Method.* (Modified from Burkitt, et al., 1972.)

Subjects	Country	Race	Type of diet	Mean transit time (hr)	Mean weight of stools passed (g)	Comments
Naval ratings and wives	U.K.	White	Refined	83.4	104	Shore-based personnel
Teenage boarding school pupils	U.K.	White	Refined	76.1	110	Institutional diet together with cakes, sweets, etc. from school shop
Students	South Africa	White	Refined	48.0	173	These ate more fruit than is usual in the U.K.
Nurses	South Africa	Indian	Mixed	44.0	155	Less refined diet than that of western world
Urban school-children	South Africa	African	Mixed	45.2	165	Partly Europeanized diet
Manor House Hospital patients	U.K.	White	Mixed	41.0	175	U.K. diet plus wholemeal bread and added bran
Senior boarding school pupils	Uganda	African	Mixed	47.0	185	Traditional Ugandan diet plus refined sugar, white bread
Vegetarians	U.K.	White	Mixed	42.4	225	Note similarity of values to those of African groups
Rural school-children	South Africa	African	Unrefined	33.5	275	
Rural villages	Uganda	African	Unrefined	35.7	470	Villagers not yet supplementing diet with processed foods of western type

*Note the inverse relationship between stool weight and transit time.

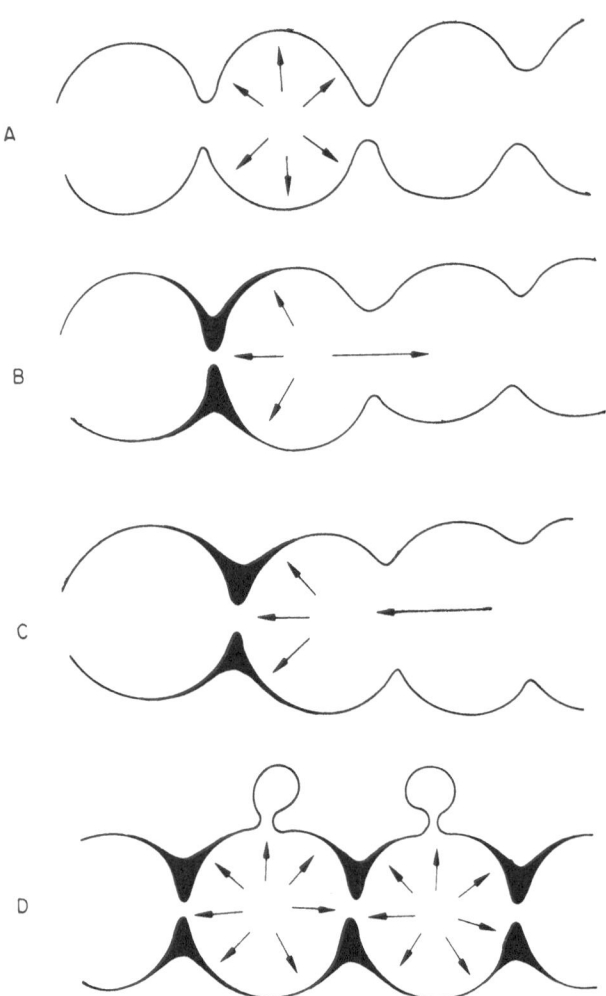

Fig. 2. The role of segmentation in colonic physiology. Diagram
shows longitudinal section of colon which has segmented so as to
localize high pressure to one segment (A). If the contraction ring
bounding this segment relaxes, its contents will flow to the right
to an area of lower pressures (B). Contraction rings can act as
"baffles" so as to halt the contents of the colon which are moving
(C). In lowest section (D) the segmented colon is acting as a
series of "little bladders" each of which harbors a high pressure.
This is how segmentation generates the pulsion force that causes
the mucosa to herniate (from Painter, 1964).

A TRIAL OF A HIGH-FIBER DIET

If it is accepted that fiber-deficiency is the cause of
diverticular disease, then the low-residue diet that has been
hallowed by usage rather than by reason, should be contraindicated
in the treatment of the disease. Furthermore, it becomes obvious
that a high-fiber diet should be tried in the treatment of symptomatic diverticular disease. This was done at Manor House Hospital
beginning in 1967. Seventy unselected patients were advised to
eat wholemeal (not brown) bread, Kelloggs' All Bran, Weetabix,
Shredded Wheat and porridge. They were asked to add miller's bran
to their diet three times a day. Each was told of the connection
between diet and diverticulosis and that bran would make their
stools soft so that their bowels did not have to contract excessively and thereby cause pain. Each was given a sheet of
instructions pointing out that bran is difficult to take when dry
and that it should be washed down with water, milk or fruit juice,
added to breakfast cereals, or taken in soup. They began by
taking one teaspoon three times a day and were told to increase
this dose after two weeks until they defecated without effort
once or twice a day. If they did not have to strain to pass a
stool, it is reasonable to deduce that their sigmoid had not
needed to segment excessively in order to propel its contents.

Patients were warned that they might feel distended or full of
air when they first took bran but that these symptoms would disappear in about two weeks with continued use of bran. They also
were told that they might have to take several tablespoons of bran
to achieve this effect. All were asked to reduce their intake of
refined sugar, whether brown or white, because refined sugar does
not occur in nature as an isolated substance and does not contain
plant fiber. Before this "Bran Diet" was prescribed, all patients
had been examined by barium enema and sigmoidoscopy to exclude any
organic stenosis of the colon. Those with stenosis due to fibrosis
were treated surgically.

Of the 70 patients, three reported that their symptoms had
disappeared on wholemeal bread and All-Bran and so they did not
take unprocessed bran. Sixty-two patients took bran regularly for
a minimum of six months and some of these subjects have now been
followed for seven years. They found that the average dose of
miller's bran was six teaspoons a day (about 12-14 g of bran containing about 2 g of cereal fiber). Some needed several tablespoons of bran daily and each found the amount required by trial
and error.

One of the remaining five patients came to surgery and it was
found that his myenteric plexus had been destroyed, probably by
taking senna for twenty years. Two of the remaining four sought

advice elsewhere and the other two did not like bran and were made
comfortable with Normacol® (Movicol®).

Most bran in England is bought at Health Stores. Almost two-
thirds of the patients felt distended when they first took bran
but this discomfort disappeared in two to three weeks. Of 57
patients queried as to their appetite, 30 had a good appetite which
was unchanged by bran; 26 had their appetite improved once they
were established on bran, and one whose appetite was poor following
a partial gastrectomy said that it remained poor after bran. In no
patient did bran make the appetite worse. This gives the lie to
the widely held belief that "roughage irritates the gut". Three
patients who had been on a low-residue diet had poor appetites and
symptoms that were improved by bran. None would return to a low-
residue diet.

As regards the need for laxatives, no less than 49 of the 70
had taken laxatives when first seen. Twenty-seven bought these at
their own expense, often spending money that they could ill afford.
Of the 62 who took bran regularly, only seven needed laxatives
and then only occasionally. Obviously, the widespread use of bran
would save patients' money and also public funds.

The symptoms of diverticulosis vary from vague dyspeptic
complaints, such as nausea, heartburn, flatulence, distension, to
lower abdominal aches and severe colic. (Table 2) Some patients
also have symptoms that are referred to the rectum, namely, a tender
rectum, constipation, and a feeling that their rectum is never
empty. The 70 patients complained of 171 symptoms, 14 of which
belonged to the eight individuals who did not take bran. Only six
(3.8%) of these symptoms were not reduced by taking bran; 62
(39.5%) were relieved and 89 (56.7%) were completely abolished by
the bran diet. Those who did not tolerate bran were made comfortable
with Normacol (Movicol) which is the best alternative to bran
since it has not been known to clump and cause obstruction. This
complication has been reported after the use of other bulk-formers.
Hence, the addition of fiber to the diet in the form of wheat bran
will relieve over 88% of the symptoms of diverticular disease. The
low-residue diet is contraindicated since it is the cause of
diverticulosis.

EPISODES OF "DIVERTICULITIS"

Bran does not abolish "diverticulitis". Two patients who were
taking bran were hospitalized for severe pain in the left iliac
fossa. Neither had evidence of true inflammatory diverticulitis
and were diagnosed as suffering from "Painful Diverticular Disease"
(Painter, 1968). With conservative treatment, both recovered.

TABLE 2. Presenting Symptoms of Seventy Patients with Diverticular Disease

	Before bran	Bran not tolerated	Symptoms after bran		
			Not relieved	Relieved	Abolished
Dyspeptic symptoms					
Nausea	11	1	1	2	7
Heartburn	2	—	—	2	—
Flatulence	2	—	1	1	—
Distension	36	4	2	14	16
Wind	13	—	—	4	9
Painful diverticular disease					
Right iliac fossa, pain or ache	7	—	—	5	2
Left iliac fossa, pain or ache	22	1	1	7	13
Lower or general abdominal pain	28	3	—	11	14
Severe colic	12	1	—	4	7
Bowel symptoms					
Tender rectum	4	—	—	1	3
Incomplete emptying of rectum	6	—	—	3	3
Constipation	28	4	1	8	15
Total	171	14	6	62	89

(from Painter, et al., 1972)

Another patient had true diverticulitis while taking bran and
responded to antibiotics and supportive therapy. All three have
taken bran since these attacks.

One patient had very severe "left renal colic" for which she
was investigated by intravenous pyelography with negative findings.
Later, diverticula were demonstrated in her colon and she was given
bran. She has suffered no further attacks but sometimes she has
an ache in the same position and with the same radiation as her
previous pain. This is mild and disappears if she increases her
intake of bran for two days. Thus, even recurrent episodes of
colic which would have led to surgery from so-called "diverticulitis" can be relieved by adding fiber to the diet.

Twelve patients of the 62 suffered from recurring attacks of
lower abdominal pain, eleven responded to the bran diet and another
to Normacol . None has come to surgery, although initially they
were all potential candidates for sigmoid resection. The widespread
adoption of the high-fiber diet would lessen the need for surgery
in diverticular disease provided that previous attacks of diverticulitis have not led to fibrosis and irreversible narrowing of the
colonic lumen.

THE ORIGIN OF THE SYMPTOMS THAT OFTEN ACCOMPANY COLONIC DIVERTICULOSIS

If it is accepted that a fiber-depleted diet can so damage the
colon that it literally "ruptures" itself, then is it not most
unlikely that the colon, and frequently only its sigmoid portion,
is the only part of the intestinal tract to be affected adversely
by this diet? The symptoms of uncomplicated diverticular disease
cannot be due to the diverticula, which are not removed when these
symptoms are abolished by bran or by Reilly's operation. Furthermore, it is difficult to attribute such "upper intestinal" symptoms
as heartburn, nausea and distension to a colonic disease. Hence,
is it not possible that the dyspepsia and abdominal discomfort
that are associated so often with diverticular disease are caused
by a dysfunction of the entire alimentary tract occasioned by its
having to struggle with a low-residue diet?

That cereal fiber affects the human bowel profoundly can be
confirmed by any doctor who is prepared to take bran himself or to
prescribe it for his patients. This cheap, effective, and safe
remedy will ease constipation, hemorrhoids, and symptomatic diverticulosis. Its effect on the frequency of defecation is dramatic
and is shown in Figure 3.

The concept that diverticular disease is caused by fiber-

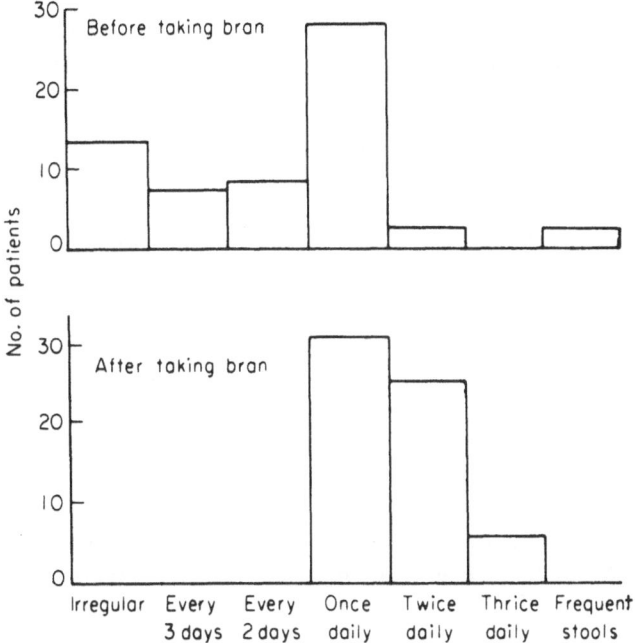

Fig. 3. Effect of unprocessed bran on the bowel habit in diverticular disease (from Painter, et al., 1972).

depletion brought about by food refining holds out the hope that this disease, like scurvy, is preventable and that it need not appear in future generations.

REFERENCES

Arfwidsson, S., 1964, Pathogenesis of multiple diverticula of the sigmoid colon in diverticular disease, Acta. Chir. Scand., 342:1-68.

Bland-Sutton, J., 1920, Discussion of secondary deposits in bone mistaken for primary tumors, Section of Surgery, Proc. Roy. Soc. Med., 13:1-5.

Burkitt, D. P., Walker, A. R. P. and Painter, N. S., 1972, Effect of dietary fiber on stools and transit times and its role in causation of disease, Lancet ii:1408-1411.

Painter, N. S., 1962, Master of Surgery Thesis, University of London.

Painter, N. S., 1964, The aetiology of diverticulosis of the colon
    with special reference to the action of certain drugs on the
    behavior of the colon, Ann. of the Roy. Coll. Surg., England,
    34:98-119.

Painter, N. S., 1968, Diverticular disease of the colon, Brit. Med.
    J., 3:475-479.

Painter, N. S. and Burkitt, D. P., 1971, Diverticular disease of
    the colon: A deficiency disease of the Western Civilization,
    Brit. Med. J., 2:450-453.

Painter, N. S., Almeida, A. Z. and Colebourne, K. W., 1972, Unpro-
    cessed bran in treatment of diverticular disease of the colon,
    Brit. Med. J., 2:137-139.

Painter, N. S., Truelove, S. C., Ardran, G. M. and Tuckey, M.,
    1965, Segmentation and the localization of intraluminal
    pressures in the human colon, with special reference to the
    pathogenesis of colonic diverticula, Gastroenterology,
    49:169-177.

Spriggs, E. I. and Marxer, O. A., 1925, Intestinal diverticula,
    Quart. J. Med., 19:1-34.

DISCUSSION

H. M. Spiro: Do you give bran to a patient who has had a
recent attack of diverticulitis with spasm, narrowing, possibly
even a small perforation?

N. S. Painter: Once they have recovered from the acute attack
and it is decided that nothing is surgically wrong and there is no
organic stenosis, they are given bran.

G. J. Devroede: Figure 1 in the discussion that follows Dr.
Almy's paper showed what the struggle between the heretics and the
orthodox had been doing to practice in Canada. I must add that I
was a heretic prescribing a high-residue diet who was uneasy
because there has not been any controlled trial. Therefore we
initiated a controlled trial three years ago. (Table 1)

I am sorry no statistics are available because data were
compiled Monday and Tuesday by our nutritionist, Dr. J. Jobecky and
the figure was made on Wednesday (Table 2). We have presently 66
patients on the trial who have been followed for a total of 729
months. The number of visits per patient is about four, with a
range of one to nine. The patient returns every three months and
the diet is reviewed each visit.

TABLE 1. Diverticular Disease--Random Trial of Medical Management, 1974 Status

Number of patients on trial:	66
Number of months of follow-up:	729
Number of visits per patient: (1 visit every 3 months)	3.6 (mean) 1-9 (range)

The study comprised six groups of patients: patients were randomized to a low-residue diet or a high-residue diet, with or without a dietary prescription with Metamucil or a placebo. Metamucil was selected because I was impressed by Carlson's study in 1949 (Carlson & Hoelzel, 1949) demonstrating no marked decrease in diverticulosis in a group taking a high-bulk diet, and almost total disappearance of diverticula if Psyllium husks were added to the high-residue diet. In our study a low-residue diet averages 13 g. Table 3 lists the therapeutic failures.

Failures were patients who refused to return three times because they were unhappy with the program, and successful patients who returned regularly and adhered to the diet but kept complaining of symptoms on three successive visits. There were 24 failures for the placebo but only eight for the Metamucil group.

Several points must be made about the overall study. Thirty-six of the patients who were on no dietary regime (the N group) and

TABLE 2. Diverticular Disease--Random Trial of Medical Management, 1974 Status. Allocation to Treatments

Medication		Diverticulosis			Diverticulitis			All Patients		
		↑R	↓R	N	↑R	↓R	N	↑R	↓R	N
Placebo	32	9	9	8	1	1	4	10	10	12
Metamucil	34	9	8	9	3	3	2	12	11	11
Total	66	18	17	17	4	4	6	22	21	23

↑R High Crude Fiber Content ↓R Low Crude Fiber Content
N Normal

TABLE 3. Diverticular Disease--Random Trial of Medical Management, 1974 Status. Failures

Medication	↑R	↓R	N	Total
Placebo	4	5	5	14
Metamucil	3	1	4	8
Total	7	6	9	22

↑R High Crude Fiber Content ↓R Low Crude Fiber Content
N Normal

received the placebo, felt better. The best group (72%) was on the low-residue diet and a placebo. Patients with Metamucil on the other hand felt better when they were on high-residue or low-residue diets. (Table 4)

Table 5 shows the symptoms score, tabulated by the nutritionist and here we have a completely different story. First of all we note the same placebo effect: 50% of the patients who had no dietary prescription and a placebo felt better. But the best group of patients was on Metamucil and no special diet, and the worst group of patients was on a low-residue diet and a placebo: there is a complete discrepancy between the overall patients' subjective impression and the symptoms score. We have additional objective data on symptoms, colonic transit times and a questionnaire on bowel habits, but these have not yet been analyzed.

TABLE 4. Diverticular Disease--Random Trial of Medical Management, 1974 Status. Overall Patient Impression (by percentage of patients)

	Placebo			Metamucil		
	↑R	↓R	N	↑R	↓R	N
Better	17	72	36	55	60	33
Worse	34	14	36	18	30	33
Can't Tell	49	14	28	27	10	34

↑R High Crude Fiber Content ↓R Low Crude Fiber Content
N Normal

TABLE 5. Diverticular Disease--Random Trial of Medical Management, 1974 Status. Symptoms Score (by percentage of patients)

	Placebo			Metamucil		
	↑R	↓R	N	↑R	↓R	N
Better	50	17	50	27	29	63
Worse	50	34	20	19	13	--
Same	--	49	30	54	58	37

↑R High Crude Fiber Content ↓R Low Crude Fiber Content
N Normal

J. Christensen: Which is the placebo?

G. J. Decroede: Metamucil is an extract of Psyllium dispersed with dextrose. The placebo was pure dextrose given in a similar amount.

H. M. Spiro: And the controls were a high-residue diet and a low-residue diet?

G. J. Devroede: There were six groups, high-residue diet with Metamucil or placebo; no diet prescription with Metamucil or placebo; and low-residue diet with Metamucil or placebo.

M. A. Eastwood: It is interesting that countless generations of physicians from Galen to Osler have prescribed brown bread and a high-roughage diet for constipation. It would appear that the introduction of the concept of the low-fiber diet emanates from Alvarez in his "Introduction to Gastroenterology", where there is a diatribe against a high-fiber containing diet. I think that Painter's contribution has been to reverse this misconception and to encourage a return to a high-fiber diet in the treatment of diverticular disease. On the other hand, to extend the therapeutic value of bran to an etiological role makes me uneasy. Data from Painter's work show that there is a steady increase in mortality in England and Wales until the 1930's when the flattening in the curve is ascribed to the introduction of the "national loaf" which was a less refined product. Since the 1950's there has developed a marked female to male predominance. I don't know that this trend can be entirely ascribed to such a difference in diet between the female and male. Statistics from Scotland show that there is a marked difference in hospital admission rates for diverticular disease and cancer of the bowel in the different geographical

regions. In the midland valley of Scotland (Glasgow and Edinburgh)
the incidence is considerably less than in the north and far north.
If these diseases are indeed diseases of civilization the reason
for this gradient in Scotland is not immediately apparent. I
would suggest that there is certainly a great deal to be said for
the high-fiber diet as a therapeutic regimen, but I feel less
confident of the etiological factors. I wonder whether there is
in fact a spasmogen in the bowel which has been diluted by the
high-fiber and the associated water retention within the bowel.

I. Williams: My comment derives from the bias of a radiologist
looking at a very obvious artefact--the colon distended almost as
far as it is able to go. When you compare an operative specimen
with its radiological counterpart, you can see that the diameter of
the colon is not really decreased in the affected segment but
approximates the diameter of each end of the unaffected bowel.
If you wish to regard the indentations as some disturbance of
circular muscle contraction, then it is necessary to design some
mechanism whereby one-third of the circular muscle around the
lumen can contract while leaving the remaining two-thirds of the
circumference relaxed. This situation is not really explicable in
terms of current ideas of electrical activity. So I think that
this pattern derives mainly from a shortening of the longitudinal
muscle which produces an accordion-like effect. The radiological
picture is a manifestation of distension, and this pattern is not
seen in the contracted colon or undistended operative specimen.
Perhaps this is why you do not see it in your hospital.

What we must identify is some particular pathology that affects
the longitudinal muscle more than the circular muscle and this
applies especially to the so-called diverticulosis, where the
pathologists find no muscular abnormality although the pattern is
present radiologically. So far, no one seems to have described any
good histological criteria for the muscular abnormality.

A. M. Connell: May I comment on one point which Ifor Williams
made about the pathological features. The electrical impulse
primarily is generated in the longitudinal muscle and in some way
spreads into the circular muscle. This might place the early
pathogenesis of the disease at a point where we could recognize
some fundamental, physiological principle. We must think in terms
of how we are affecting the longitudinal muscle of the alimentary
tract. I have been de-emphasizing the motility changes, partly
because I feel that the simplistic view of the etiology of diverticular disease does not really explain all the features of the
disease. What we are seeing may be effects on muscle which are
derived from other mechanisms and from other locales in the
alimentary tract. One of the great benefits of this meeting has
been to bring into the open the many variables in this situation

in the hope that our discussion will lead us toward thinking of other possibile mechanisms.

R. W. Wissler: My interests in fiber consumption actually are focused more on its relation to heart disease than to gastro-intestinal disease. We are not covering this topic today, but I would like to point out that Dr. David Kritchevsky presented an excellent review of this subject entitled "Nonnutritive and lipid metabolism", May 14, 1974, at the Meeting of Institute of Food Technologists (Kritchevsky & Storey, 1974). His co-author, John Storey, is here today and might wish to comment.

I am not quite as pessimistic as Dr. Dietschy about the probable results of more fiber in the diet. Recently, I spent two months in Japan, studying coronary heart disease and, anec-dotally at least, the Japanese diet. The Japanese have a low incidence of both atherosclerosis and coronary heart disease, even in these modern times in highly urbanized Tokyo. I suspect that this situation may have more to do with fiber in the Japanese diet than with a low consumption of eggs, meat, or other foods high in saturated fats and cholesterol.

I also would like to make a few comments about chenodeoxy-cholic acid. Two days ago, I attended a very interesting meeting on comparative pathology at the Armed Forces Institute of Pathology. Professor Tom Clarkson of Bowman-Gray University described his work with squirrel monkeys fed graded step-wise doses of cheno-deoxycholic acid. He found that the greater the amount of acid included in the mixed synthetic diet with cholesterol and saturated fat (in this case, lard), the greater was the tendency for these animals to develop cirrhosis. Therefore, I think that we should be somewhat cautious in extolling the beneficial aspects of fiber-containing diets that raise the level of chenodeoxycholic acid in the bowel. The health of the liver also must be kept in mind.

Clarkson has also been working with another type of monkey, Macaca nemestrina, in experiments relating to atherosclerosis. On a highly-saturated, low-fiber, cholesterol-containing diet, these animals manifested a very high incidence of cirrhosis of the liver. There is some preliminary evidence that this also may be due to the toxic effects of chenodeoxycholic acid or one of its derivatives absorbed from the gut. The senior author on the squirrel monkey study is Abbey, and his work will be published in the near future. It provides a note of caution about some of the bile acid effects which should concern us in fiber studies. I do not think that Dr. Burkitt included the incidence of cirrhosis on his very interesting maps, but it generally tends to show an increase in frequency in those areas where carcinoma of the colon, atherosclerosis and diverticulosis are at low frequency.

REFERENCES

Carlson, A. J., Hoelzel, F., 1949, Relation of diet to diverticu-
     losis in rats, Gastroenterology, 12:108-115.

Kritchevsky, D., and Storey, J. A., 1974, Binding of bile salts
     in vitro by non-nutritive fiber, J. Nutr., 104:458-462.

SURGICAL ASPECTS OF DIVERTICULAR DISEASE

A. N. Smith

Gastrointestinal Unit, Western General Hospital

Edinburgh, Scotland

Diverticular disease of the colon has been described as a disease of Western civilization and its causation attributed to a deficiency of dietary fiber by Painter (1970). Most patients who have operations for diverticular disease nowadays have had a preliminary period of management on a high-fiber diet or a hydrophilic colloid, both of which produce bulkier fecal residues. The latter was shown by Hodgson (1972) to produce a lowering of intraluminal colonic pressures. If excessive intraluminal pressure, as emphasized by Arfwidsson (1964) and Painter (1964) is the important factor in the genesis of diverticular disease, it follows that operations for diverticular disease may have to be judged on their ability to reduce this abnormality. As a consequence, some assessment of the length of time for which the operative change is effective would be valuable. Possibly beneficial changes could easily lapse if the patients continued to be exposed after operation to the same conditions as those obtaining before operation.

It is important first to define the effect of the common operations performed for diverticular disease in terms of motility and to determine how long the effects last in patients continuing on their original diet, compared with others given supplementary fiber, such as bran, post-operatively. In this respect, it is also opportune to try to gauge the efficacy of the newer operation of colo-myotomy compared with the standard operation of "resection and anastomosis" usually performed for gross diverticular disease.

In recent years there has been a shift in emphasis from inflammation to the "thick muscle syndrome" in diverticular disease following the description of this by Morson (1963) and Watts and

Marcus (1964). Reilly (1966) in England has described an operation
of longitudinal colo-myotomy which was intended to deal rationally
with the thick muscle, the high pressure produced, and the direct
obstructive effects of this situation. A third operation has
been described which takes into account Williams' idea regarding
the importance of the taeniae in this condition: Hodgson and
Johnson have been dividing the taeniae as their form of "transverse
taeniomyotomy" (Hodgson, 1973; Johnson, 1972).

EFFECTS OF LONGITUDINAL MYOTOMY AND
RESECTION UPON MOTILITY

Here I shall compare and contrast the effects of Reilly's
longitudinal myotomy with resection and anastomosis in terms of
motility. The patients examined were subjects with uncomplicated
diverticular disease, studied on their habitual diet before and
after the addition of bran, and then selected for operation on the
basis of a high pre-operative intraluminal pressure, as recorded
manometrically. They were a selected group and not part of any
other trial; the myotomy patients were mainly a rather older
group often with severe concomitant disease such as ischemic heart
disease, or emphysema. They only underwent a myotomy if a thick
colonic muscle could be demonstrated. Transit times were studied
using "Hinton" markers (Hinton, et al., 1969) and the motility was
recorded by standard technics (Smith, 1971b).

In uncomplicated diverticular disease there is excessive
activity following intake of food or administration of neostigmine
and this is lessened in each case by colo-myotomy (Attisha & Smith,
1969). Our experiments showed that there was no significant
increase in the basal mean motility index (Figure 1) which implies
that the circular muscle may be thick but does not act significantly
at rest. In diverticular disease, food produces a much greater
mean motility index than in normal subjects; but after myotomy the
index returns to approximately normal levels. Neostigmine produced
an excessive effect in patients with diverticular disease and this
too was reduced to normal levels by myotomy.

The statistical treatment of this information shows no change
in the basal state; the food-provoked reflex was reduced by
myotomy, and the change after neostigmine was reduced to normal
levels by colo-myotomy at two to three months after operation.
This decrease was maintained after one year of observation.
(Table 1)

In comparison, the resection patients, as Parks (1970) has
also shown demonstrated no comparable response to myotomy following
food stimulation and after neostigmine. The change in motor

TABLE 1. Post-myotomy of Pelvic Colon (14 patients); Mean Motility Indices Compared with Normals (9 volunteers) and Diverticular Disease (29 patients) in the Resting State after Food and after a Cholinergic Stimulus

	Normals	Diverticular Disease	After Sigmoid Myotomy
Basal activity	151	343	130
	No significant difference in the groups ($0.3 < P < 0.2$)		
Gastrocolic reflex	263 Significant increase ($P < 0.001$)	740 Significantly higher than normals ($P < 0.001$)	347 Significantly reduced after myotomy ($P = 0.01$) No difference from normals ($0.4 > P > 0.3$)
After prostigmine	791 Significant increase ($P = 0.001$)	2856 Significantly higher than normals ($P < 0.001$)	1183 Significantly reduced after myotomy ($P = 0.001$) No difference from normals ($0.4 > P > 0.3$)

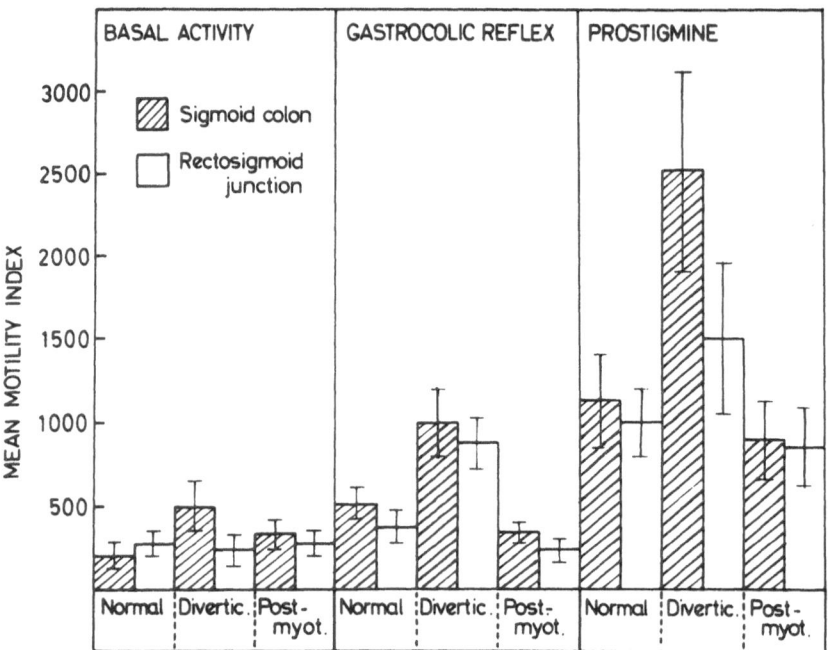

Fig. 1.   The mean motility index (± SE) for normals, diverticular
disease and post-myotomy cases: the records were taken in a
resting period, after food and after a cholinergic stimulus from
the sigmoid and rectosigmoid levels.

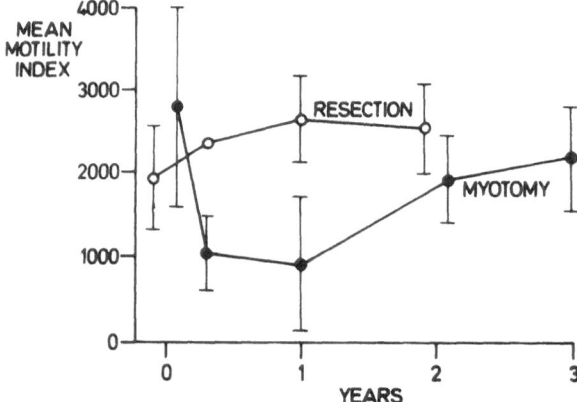

Fig. 2.   The motility index in a group of 12 myotomy and resection
cases is compared at 3 months, 1, 2 and 3 years.

activity of the bowel appears to be a generalized rather than a localized effect. Table 2 indicates that the motility level was still significantly above normal (Smith, et al., 1971a). This was true for a food stimulus as well as for a cholinergic one.

A further follow-up of the colo-myotomy patients was conducted for two and three years (Smith, et al., 1971b). The initial effect of colo-myotomy was a period of reduced pressure which lasted for about a year after which the pressures started to rise during the second or third year. In comparison, the resection group maintained a pressure at or slightly above the pre-operative level throughout. (Figure 2)

EFFECTS OF POST-OPERATIVE ADMINISTRATION OF BRAN

Since so many of these patients had been on a regime with a high-fiber intake with bran or with hydrophilic colloid agents, we decided that we must consider the need for these agents post-operatively, especially in regard to the possibility of inducing a more protracted or effective reduction of the intraluminal pressure in the colon. Many of the patients who experienced a return of high intracolonic pressures apparently could soon be symptomatic again and it was opportune to discover how relevant was their post-operative maintenance on a high-fiber intake.

A group of patients with diverticular disease was first compared with normal subjects while being given a course of 20 g of unprocessed bran daily in addition to their diet for one month (Findlay, et al., 1974). The reduction in transit time in diver-

TABLE 2. Mean Motility Indices after Neostigmine Stimulation in 12 Patients with Local Obstruction and Thickened Musculature before and after Resection of the Pelvic Colon (12 of the 20 cases were suitable in age, etc. for comparison with Table 1)

Mean motility index ($\pm$SD)		
Normals	Pre-resection	Post-resection (at 3/12)
791 $\pm$ 102	1468 $\pm$ 850	1891 $\pm$ 480
	Still significantly increased above normal after resection.	
	$P < 0.001$	

TABLE 3.   Diverticular Disease: Pre- Post-Bran: 9 Patients

	Pre-bran	Post-bran	Change
		Transit Time (hrs)	
Normals	66.3±18.1	50.0±11.5	-14.7±10.9
Divertic.	93.4±13.8	57.9±8.0	-36.9±7.0 (P < 1%)

ticular disease was much greater than in normal subjects. (Table 3)
In nine patients who were their own controls there was a reduction
in pressure insignificant in regard to the basal level.   Pressure
was significantly reduced after prostigmine, and to a relatively
greater degree in respect of the gastro-colic reflex in that it
fell to levels lower than the basal state.   (Figure 3)

This observation supported the plan for the use of bran during
the post-operative period and this was done five years ago, after

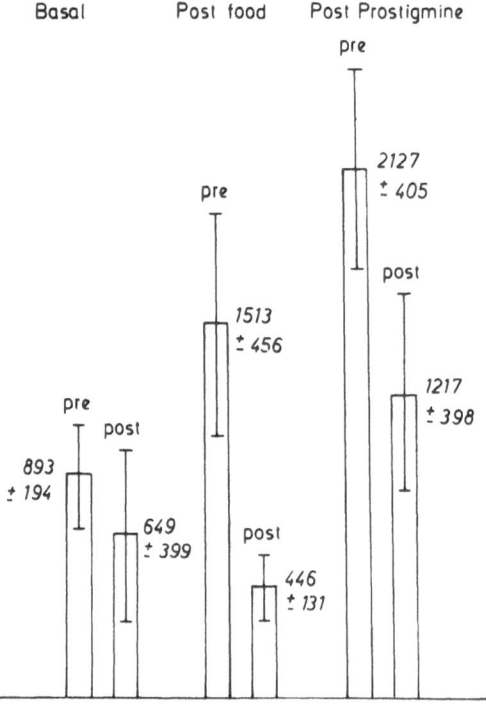

Fig. 3.   Colonic motility activity in 9 diverticular disease
patients before and after bran.

the third Gastrointestinal Motility Meeting when Painter described
his studies of patients with diverticular disease (Burkitt, et al.,
1972).

Five post-operative patients were put on bran and compared
over five years with patients managed by resection and anastomosis
without bran. (Figure 4a) The group without bran maintained a
high pressure throughout the five-year period as they were studied
at three months, two, three, four, and five years. In contrast,
the five similar patients on 20 g of bran daily showed a reduction
in pressure over this period. There was an even greater reduction
in the myotomy patients taking bran (Figure 4b) in comparison with
the non-bran group who showed a tendency to return to high pressure
levels after the initial reduction. After bran, the pressures were
maintained at such low levels that even myotomy patients who had
been subjected to what might be considered as a very modified
surgical procedure were not in danger of developing complications
from returning intracolonic pressures.

In summary, 20 g of bran per day shortens the intestinal

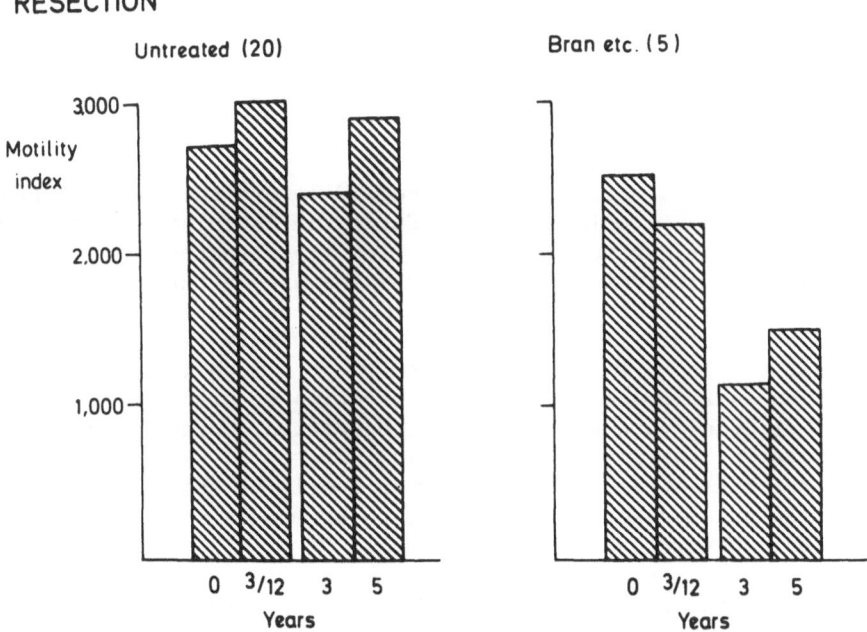

Fig. 4a. The mean motility indices in 20 resection cases are shown
over 4-5 years. In five comparable cases given tests at similar
intervals but put on bran after their resection there was a fall in
motility (15 tests P<0.01).

MYOTOMY

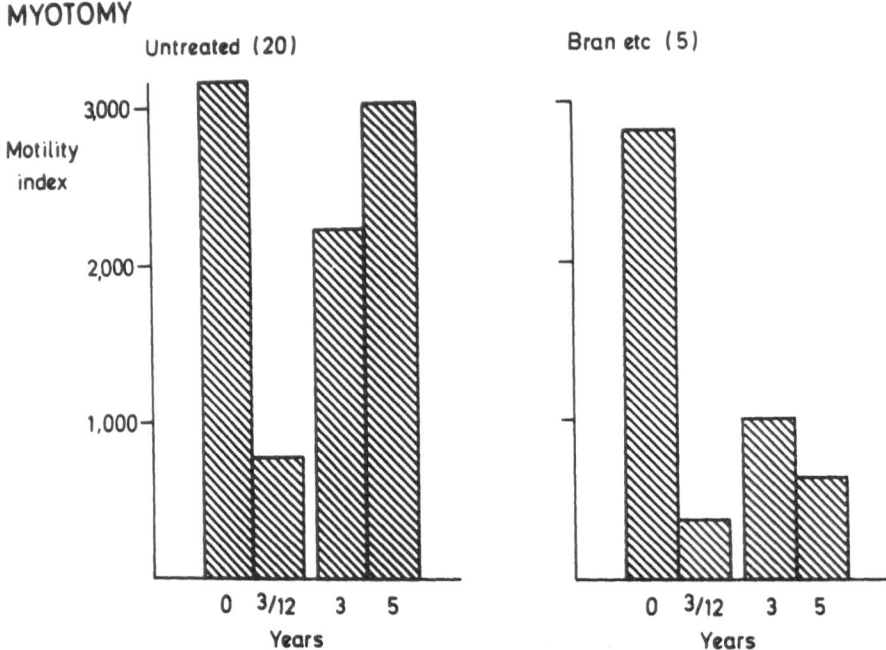

Fig. 4b. After myotomy in five comparable patients there was also a significant reduction. Comparisons of the effect in the 3-5 year period with and without bran when the myotomy group had a return of pressure showed an even more significant effect (p<0.005).

transit time in diverticular disease and lowers the intraluminal pressure. Sigmoid colo-myotomy reduces the intraluminal pressure but the pressures return post-operatively over three to five years. The intraluminal pressure remains high after resection of the pelvic colon for diverticular disease, and seems to implicate the colonic muscle in an abnormality more widely situated than in the pelvic colon. The pressures remain at a much lower level if operation is followed by the administration of bran. An important aspect of colo-myotomy is that this operation, which initially is effective in lowering the intraluminal pressure, emphasizes the important role played by the circular muscle of the colon in diverticular disease. The thick circular muscle occasionally can be almost obstructive in its action.

In a surgical follow-up of 30 myotomy patients who have been treated by this operation in Edinburgh there was one death, and this was of a patient who was a severe asthmatic receiving steroids and who experienced perforation of the colon post-operatively. (Table 4) Some of these patients not on bran now have had a

TABLE 4.   Myotomy Results

Number	30 Cases	
Gross morbidity	2 Pelvic abcess ⎨ 1 jaundice / 1 with fistula	
Technique	1 Longitudinal myotomy 4 Proximal colostomy 15 Temporary tube cecostomy 2 Proximal exteriorisation 9 Myotomy alone	
Assessment (27)	Radiology	9 Diverticula 'reduced' 10 Formerly, not now, 'obstructed' 7 Wider 1 Stricture
	Motility	Reduced in all except 'stricture'
(25)	Clinical	17 Symptom free (5 on bran; not included) 3 recurrent symptoms→/re-operation
	Deaths	1 Operative: 4 late; concurrent diseases

recurrence of their symptoms; the five patients who have been maintained on this therapeutic measure are to date symptom-free.

REFERENCES

Attisha, R. P. and Smith, A. N., 1969, Pressure activity of the colon and rectum in diverticular disease before and after sigmoid myotomy, Brit. J. Surg., 56:891-894.

Arfwidsson, S., Kock, N. C., Lehman, L., 1964, Pathogenesis of multiple diverticula of the colon in diverticular disease, Acta Chir. Scand. Suppl., 342:1-68.

Findlay, J. M., Smith, A. N., Mitchell, W. D., Anderson, A. J. B. and Eastwood, M. A., 1974, Effects of unprocessed bran on colon function in normal subjects and in diverticular disease, Lancet, i:146-148.

Hinton, J. M., Lennard-Jones, J. E. and Young, A. C., 1969, Gut, 10:842-847.

Hodgson, J., 1972, Effect of methyl cellulose on rectal and colonic pressure in diverticular disease, Brit. Med. J., 3:729-731.

Hodgson, W. J. B., 1973, Transverse taeniomyotomy for diverticular disease, Dis. Colon Rectum, 16:283.

Johnson, A. G., 1972, The effect of transverse section of the taeniae coli (taeniomyotomy) on intracolonic pressure in the rabbit, Scand. J. of Gastroent., 7:321-327.

Morson, B. C., 1963, The muscle abnormality in diverticular disease of the sigmoid colon, Brit. J. Radiol., 36:385-392.

Painter, N. S., 1964, The aetiology of diverticulosis of the colon with special reference to the action of certain drugs on the behavior of the colon, Ann. Roy. Coll. Surg. Eng., 34:98-119.

Painter, N. S., 1970, Diverticular disease: a disease of this century, D. M. Publications, June:3-57.

Painter, N. S., Personal communication, subsequently, Burkitt, D. P., Walker, A. R. P., and Painter, N. S., 1972, Effect of dietary fiber in stools and transit times and its role in the causation of disease, Lancet, ii:1408-1411.

Parks, T. G., Rectal and colonic studies after resection of the colon for diverticular disease, 1970, Gut, 11:121-125.

Reilly, M., 1966, Sigmoid myotomy, Brit. J. Surg., 53:859.

Smith, A. N., Attisha, R. P. and Clarke, S., 1971a, Motility after colo-myotomy and resection of the colon for diverticular disease, Am. J. Dig. Dis., 16:728-733.

Smith, A. N., Giannakos, V. and Clarke, S., 1971b, Late results of colo-myotomy, J. Roy. Coll. Surg. Edinb., 16:276-286.

Smith, A. N., Kirwan, W. O., and Shariff, S., The effects of operations and of bran on the colon in diverticular disease, Proc. Roy. Soc. Med. (in the press).

Watt, J., Marcus, R., 1964, The pathology of diverticulosis of the antimesenteric inter-taenial area of the pelvic colon, J. Path. Bact., 88:97-106.

DISCUSSION

H. M. Spiro: Will you please clarify the original indication
for the operations of resection or myotomy?

A. N. Smith: Uncomplicated diverticular disease. Not diverticulitis, but simply patients who had continuing obstructive
features, a high colonic pressure and a thick muscle. Some of them
in fact were operated on because they also had a palpable mass and
it seemed important to rule out carcinoma. These patients, at
operation, had a thick bobbin-like mass of muscle involving the
pelvic colon.

H. M. Spiro: So you are saying that though the pressures go
down for two years, they again rise unless bran is given post-
operatively. I find myself a little uncertain as to whether I
would want these patients operated on at all or whether I would
simply put them on bran.

A. N. Smith: We have studied a separate group of patients on
bran alone without surgery. In spite of the efficacy of bran,
there are still some patients who need operations. There were,
after all, failures in Painter's trial. But some people have such
a degree of obstruction caused by the thick bands of muscle in the
pelvic colon that they require an operation. In Britain, the most
usual approach at present is to select patients for surgery on the
basis of their response to a period of trial on a hydrophilic
colloid or bran. But I would repeat that colo-myotomy also may
be a temporary measure, and all our patients so managed now receive
bran post-operatively. This seems to be essential to perpetuate
the effect.

N. S. Painter: Regarding Dr. Eastwood's remarks on the crude
death rate in England, this would have been higher after rationing
of foods ceased in 1952 had it not been for advances in surgery,
anaesthetics and antibiotics. This improvement began with
Smithwick (1942). The death rate of women may have risen more
after the war because the men were dying of lung cancer and coronary disease. Furthermore, women will not eat bread because it is
said to be fattening.

I think Dr. Smith's work on myotomy and colonic pressure is
most important. Myotomy cuts the circular muscle and widens the
bowel lumen so that the pressures decline. Parks (Proc. Roy. Soc.
Med., 1969) showed that only 65% of patients were free of symptoms
after resection for diverticulitis. These patients had returned
to a low-residue diet. Michael Reilly and Owen Daniels, a surgeon

in Wales, did about 100 myotomies on their patients and found that over 90% of them remained symptom free. This satisfactory result was due at least in part to the fact that both these surgeons returned their patients to a high-fiber diet. This would keep the pressures down and avoid return of symptoms, judging from Adam Smith's findings.

In the case of an aniline dye worker with a papilloma of the urinary baldder, his contact with the dye would be discontinued after operation. Similarly, in this disease the cause would be avoided by putting all patients on a high-fiber diet post-operatively. Otherwise, subjects who have a resection at 45 and then go back on a low-residue diet may need another resection later in life. Finally, one hears much about the irritable colon; 60% of patients attending a gastrointestinal clinic are said to have symptoms caused by an irritable gut. I do not believe that 60% of the population are born with abnormal intestines. Since the condition usually responds to a high-fiber diet we should talk of the "irritated" bowel syndrome.

FIBER-DEFICIENCY AND COLONIC TUMORS

Denis Burkitt

Medical Research Council

London, England

Most of the evidence that I shall present relating large bowel tumors, both benign and malignant, to low-fiber diets will be epidemiological. As Dr. Hegsted said this morning, epidemiological relationships do not prove anything. However, they do provide an opportunity for formulating hypotheses that subsequently can be tested, and disproved, modified, or confirmed. I shall begin by placing tumors of the colon and rectum in the context of some other diseases with which they are constantly related epidemiologically. These include medical problems of such major importance in the Western world as diverticular disease, the most prevalent disorder of the large bowel; ischemic heart disease, the commonest cause of death; gallstones, the commonest indication for abdominal surgery; hiatus hernia, which is estimated to be present in approximately 20% of the adult population; and appendicitis, which is responsible for the commonest abdominal emergency operation. All of these diseases have their highest prevalence in Western Europe and North America and their lowest in rural Africa and other similar regions (Figure 1). In contrast, the prevalence of all these diseases is comparable in black and white Americans today (Figure 2). This again contrasts with South Africa where the prevalence of these diseases in white South Africans already is similar to that of North Americans, but in total contrast to that of black South Africans (Figure 3).

WORLD DISTRIBUTION OF SOME DISEASES

We have attempted to develop maps of the world distribution of large bowel cancer, ischemic heart disease, gallstones, and

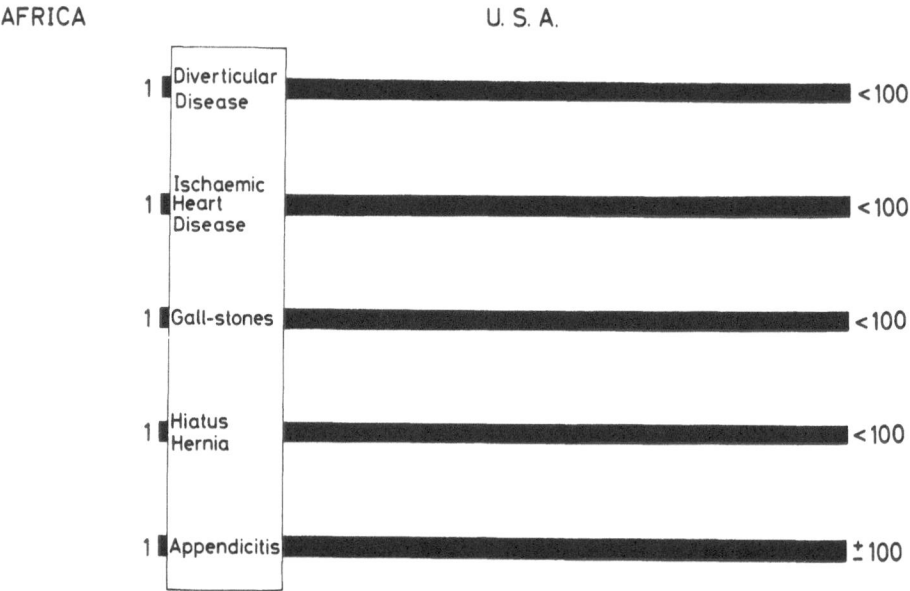

Fig. 1.   Contrasting disease prevalence in Africa and the U.S. A.

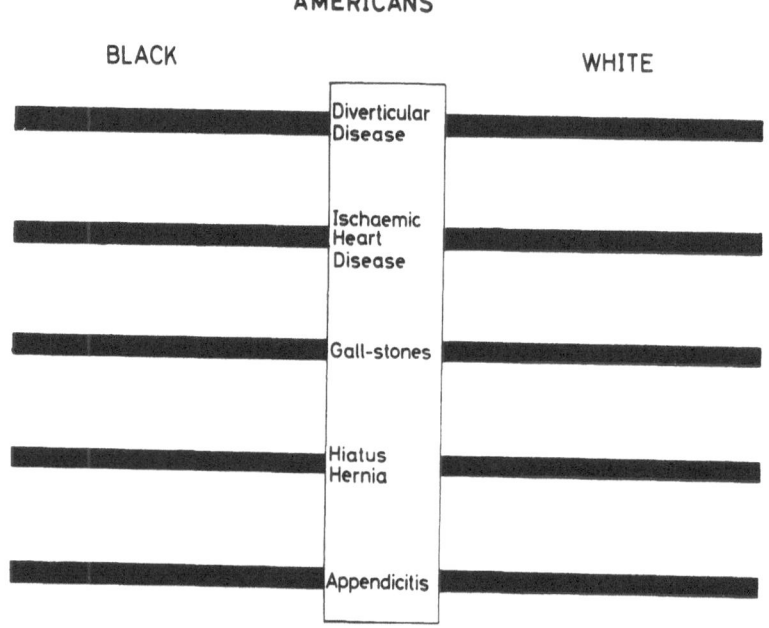

Fig. 2.   Similar disease prevalence in black and white Americans.

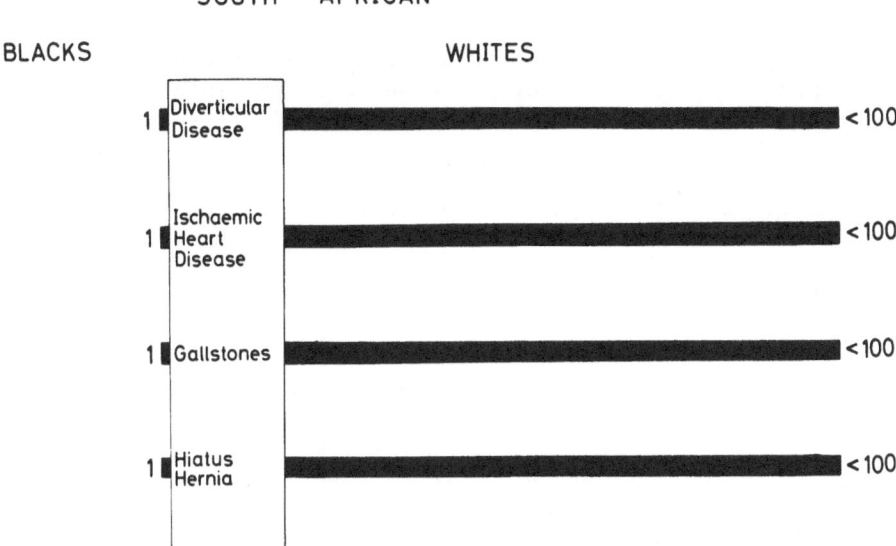

Fig. 3. Contrasting disease prevalence in black and white South Africans.

diverticular disease. We find that the distribution of each is comparable, with maximum prevalence in North Americans, both black and white, in Northern and Western Europeans, Australians and New Zealanders, and in white South Africans. The lowest prevalence is in rural Africa and in rural areas in other less economically developed countries. Intermediate prevalence rates are found in the Indian sub-continent, the Middle East and South America. Information so far is only available from certain areas, but my office receives monthly information from over 130 rural hospitals in over 30 countries, mostly in Africa and the Indian sub-continent.

The similar distribution, both geographically and in developing countries, on a socio-economic basis, suggests that some etiological factor may be common to each. Painter has outlined the evidence suggesting that diverticular disease results from a fiber-depleted diet. Heaton has presented in his book "Bile Salts in Health and Disease" (1972) the evidence pointing to fiber-depleted carbo-hydrate foods as possibly the main causative factor in the pro-duction of cholesterol gallstones, and Trowell has provided considerable evidence in support of his contention that fiber-deficient diets may be a major hitherto unconsidered factor in the pathogenesis of ischemic heart disease. The prevalence of appendicitis, in every situation examined, has risen for some decades before any appreciable rise in prevalence of any of the other diseases mentioned, and much evidence has been provided by Short, Walker and Burkitt to incriminate fiber-depleted diets in the etiology of this disease.

Other cancers of the gastrointestinal tract, such as those of the esophagus or stomach, have characteristic geographical distributions but they have nothing at all in common with the distribution of large bowel cancer and the diseases associated with it.

INFLUENCE OF DIETARY FIBER

All this information suggests that the prevalence of tumors of the large bowel might be influenced by the fiber-content of the diet, and we must postulate mechanisms whereby this might be so. Whereas alterations in the fat or protein content of the diet have not produced significant alterations in intestinal transit time and stool bulk and consistency, changes in the fiber-content of the diet alter these factors profoundly.

The inverse relationship between intestinal transit times and daily stool weights, and the relationship between these factors and the fiber-content of the diet is shown in Figure 4. Not only do transit times increase and stool weights diminish with a reduction of dietary-fiber, but the prevalence of bowel cancer and

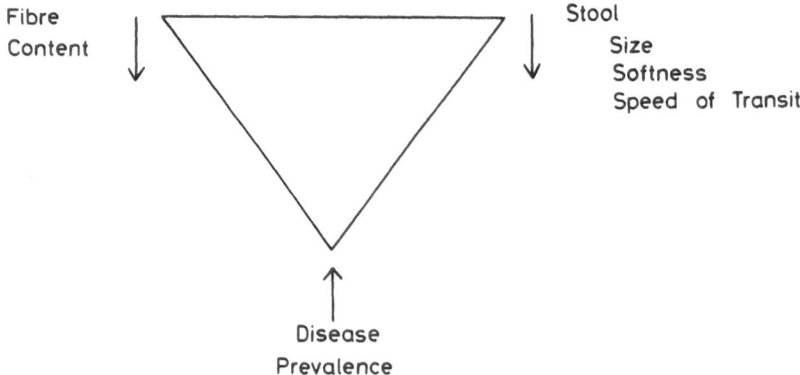

Fig. 4. Relationships between the prevalence of certain diseases, dietary fiber, and stool characteristics.

its associated diseases is related to stool bulk and consistency, and intestinal transit time.

In considering possible causative factors in bowel cancer it is significant that whereas the mucosal surface area of the small bowel is over 100 times greater than that of the large bowel, malignant tumors are more than 100 times, and benign tumors more than 1000 times commoner in the large bowel. Even taking into account the fact that the colonic mucosa may be more liable to malignant change, these observations suggest that the responsible carcinogenic factors are more likely to be formed or activated in the large bowel than to be consumed in an active form in the diet.

The possibility of bacterial activity naturally comes to mind, particularly in view of the fact that maintaining rats in a sterile environment keeps them free from bowel cancer in circumstances that will produce tumors in normal animals.

Some of the most important work yet done on the pathogenesis of bowel cancer must be that of Williams, Hill, Dresar and Aries (Hill, et al., 1971) who have shown that the bacterial flora of the feces from areas with a low prevalence of bowel cancer, such as India, Uganda and Japan, differs from that of stools from high-prevalence areas such as Britain and North America. Anaerobes capable of degrading bile acids to potentially carcinogenic substances such as deoxycholate, predominate in the stools from high-incidence areas. This evidence can be linked with the relationship between bowel cancer and transit time, and stool weights.

It is not known what dietary changes alter the spectrum of bowel bacteria. Some authorities blame fat while others blame fiber. No matter what dietary changes alter the type of bacteria in the feces, the intestinal delay associated with fiber-depleted diets might be expected to provide more time, not only for bacterial proliferation, but also for the process of degrading bile salts to potentially carcinogenic substances. Moreover, the intestinal stasis and reduction of stool bulk would greatly concentrate any carcinogens thus formed and would consequently enhance their action upon the bowel mucosa.

Whether or not this postulated mechanism of bowel carcinogenesis is correct, there is a significant relationship between the fiber-content of the diet, the speed of transit, the consistency and size of stools, and the prevalence of bowel cancer and its associated diseases (Figure 4).

In the case of ischemic heart disease and of lung cancer, we know that the associated milieu interieur is raised serum lipids and tobacco smoke in the heart and the lung, respectively. Efforts consequently are made to alter these associated environments. The milieu interieur associated with bowel cancer is that of small, hard, slowly-passing feces. This can be simply and cheaply reversed by adding fiber, and particularly cereal-fiber to the diet. This will prevent or relieve constipation. There is good evidence to suggest that it will prevent or relieve diverticular disease and hemorrhoids. It may reduce the prevalence of bowel cancer in the next generation. There is no evidence that it will do any harm.

REFERENCES

Burkitt, D. P., 1971a, Epidemiology of cancer of the colon and rectum, Cancer, 28:3-13.

Burkitt, D. P., 1971b), Some neglected leads to cancer causation, J. Natn. Cancer Inst., 47:913-919.

Burkitt, D. P., 1973, "Carcinoma of the colon and rectum", in Modern Trends in Oncology, (ed. R. W. Raven), London, Butterworths.

Burkitt, D. P. & James, P. A., 1973, Low-residue diets and hiatus hernia, Lancet, ii:128-130

Doll, R., Payne, P. and Waterhouse, J. (Eds.), 1966, Cancer Incidence in Five Continents, UICC Report, Heidelberg, Springer-Verlag.

Heaton, K. W., 1973, Food fiber as an obstacle to energy intake, Lancet, ii:1418-1421.

Heaton, K. W., 1972, Bile Salts in Health and Disease, Edinburgh, Scotland, Churchill Livingstone.

Hill, M. J., Crowther, J. S., Drasar, B. S., Hawksworth, G., Aries, V. and Williams, R. E. O., 1971, Bacteria and etiology of cancer of large bowel, Lancet, 1:95-100.

Lawrence, J. C., 1936, Gastrointestinal polyps. Statistical study of malignancy incidence, Amer. J. Surg., 31:499-505.

Morson, B. C. and Bussey, H. J. R., 1970, "Predisposing Causes of Intestinal Cancer". Current Problems in Surgery, Year Book Medical Publishers, Inc., Chicago.

Oettle, A. G., 1967, "Primary neoplasms of the alimentary canal in whites and Bantu of the Transvaal, 1949-1953. A histopathological series". In Tumors of the Alimentary Tract in Africans, Nat. Cancer Inst. Monog., 25:97-109.

Painter, N. S., 1964, The etiology of diverticulosis of the colon with special reference to the action of certain drugs on the behavior of the colon, Ann. Roy. Coll. Surg. Eng., 34:98-119.

Painter, N. S. and Burkitt, D. P., 1971, Diverticular disease of the colon: A deficiency disease of Western civilization, Brit. Med. J., 2:450-454.

Quinland, W. S. and Cuff, J. R., 1940, Primary carcinoma in the negro, Arch. Path., 30:393-402.

Ringertz, N., 1967, "Epidemiology of Gastrointestinal Cancers in Scandinavia. I. Report on Denmark, Finland, Norway and Sweden". In Tumors of the Alimentary Tract in Africans, Nat. Cancer Inst. Monog., 25:219-239.

Stemmermann, G. N., 1970, Patterns of disease among Japanese living in Hawaii, Arch. Environ. Health, 20:266-273.

DISCUSSION

A. I. Mendeloff: Dr. Burkitt of course, has stimulated much of this discussion and all I can do is repeat something about his own work and then try to show wherein we have data, some of which I have been able to gather myself in recent years, to either support or make it less likely that we are talking about the same thing. In Table 1, I list the diseases that Dr. Burkitt has postulated as influenced by low-fiber intake.

TABLE 1. Fiber Epidemiology. Dr. Denis Burkitt postulates that low fiber intake increases the incidence of the following.

1. Appendicitis
2. Diverticulosis coli
3. Polyps of the colon
4. Cancer of the colon
5. Hemorrhoids
Other workers would add
6. Duodenal ulcer

TABLE 2. Patients with Acute Appendicitis as a Proportion of
Total Discharges. Five PAS Hospitals in Four Michigan Cities,
January 1960-December 1969.

Biennium	Total Discharges[1]	Patients with Acute Appendicitis[2]	
		Number	Percent
1960-1961	77,405	1,337	1.7
1962-1963	81,102	1,319	1.6
1964-1965	91,227	1,358	1.5
1966-1967	86,718	1,199	1.4
1968-1969	86,276	1,217	1.4

[1]Excludes obstetric and newborn discharges
[2]Final diagnosis explaining admission of ICDA 550.0, 550.1, or
H-ICDA 540.0, or 540.1
(from Wylie & Holly, 1972)

In the last two years I have been particularly involved in
collecting data on digestive diseases in the United States.
Table 2 demonstrates dynamic trends in the past five years.

The incidence of appendicitis in this country has decreased
40% in 20 years, perhaps more. But in every study on a localized
population, the incidence is decreasing at an extraordinary rate,
exceeded only by the declining rate of duodenal ulcer. So, the
acute appendicitis postulated by Dr. Burkitt to be a disease
involved with low-fiber intake, seems to be decreasing at a very
rapid rate while cancer of the colon is maintaining its level and
actually increasing. On the other hand pancreatic cancer is
increasing steadily. This trend has nothing to do with the
concepts discussed today. We concede that fiber has something
important to offer here but we do not know whether it is the
amount of fiber, the kind of fiber, the fact that when you eat
fiber you do not eat something else and so on.

With respect to cancer, the National Cancer Institute since
1935 has maintained very careful autopsy studies on all American
Indians. The latest publication, November 1973, points out that
in an Indian group with an overall incidence of cancer approximately
two-thirds that of whites, figures for cancer of the colon and
rectum are now the same as among American whites. Of course,
American Indians have a marked increase in cancer of the gallbladder, salivary glands, uterus and cervix in women, and greatly
lower rates for cancer of the lung, breast and bladder, particularly in males. Here then is a group that has a dietary intake

quite different from that of the rest of the United States, but has apparently a very similar rate of cancer of the colon.

The next question I would like to ask Dr. Burkitt is why the death rates for cancer of the colon in Finland, the country which has the highest rate of ischemic heart disease deaths in the world, is so low. The incidence of cancer of the colon in Finland is nine per hundred thousand, similar to that of Japan. The Finns eat very large amounts of fat and protein. How much fiber they eat, I don't know, but their cancer rates whould compare with those for the West. In fact, for colonic cancer, they do not.

One clinical point must be raised: What is the correlation between a history of constipation and the development of cancer of the colon? So far as I can tell, it is totally negative. It is impossible to demonstrate that people who develop cancer of the colon have shown any significant incidence of constipation. It is not true that people with diverticular disease, for example, have a higher incidence of cancer of the colon. So, in considering these various points which are legitimate outgrowths of Dr. Burkitt's views on dietary fiber, one would like answers that are consistent with his concept of contact time, transit time, etc., as well as the dietary habits of population groups. I, therefore, would caution against making broad statements about the total incidence of any disease in a country. I have studied very carefully the publications of the Atomic Bomb Casualty Commission in Japan, where the Hiroshima and Nagasaki death rates have been observed since 1946. Two cities more different in their disease pattern would be hard to imagine. You would not think they were in the same country, yet they are only 100 miles apart.

As Dr. Burkitt pointed out, cancer of the stomach has an extremely irregular distribution. The United States now has the lowest incidence of cancer of the stomach of any country of the world. It is extremely difficult to understand why in this country, death rates for every disease are much higher on both Coasts than in the Southwest. All death rates for the United States are lower in the Southwestern and South Central areas than on either coast. The Northeast has rates which are higher than the Southeast but both coastal areas have high death rates generally. I am sure that the fiber story contains many important clues; I think they have to be approached by direct and specific studies.

REFERENCES

Wylie, C. M., Holly, T. L., 1972, Is appendicitis increasing in the U.S. population?, PAS Reporter, 10:p.2.

PART IV
GENERAL DISCUSSION

GENERAL DISCUSSION

D. P. Burkitt: I am very interested, naturally, in the
decreased incidence of appendicitis in the United States, and I
would like to indicate immediately that I believe all of the
conditions we have been discussing have multiple etiologic factors,
of which fiber-deficient diets are only one.   There is satisfactory
anatomical and pathological evidence to explain the pathogenesis
of appendicitis on the basis of stasis of feces and hard feces.
It is a difficult problem but Mr. Tovey and I are working dili-
gently on it.

The question of the Pima Indians is interesting because they
are very prone to develop gallstones and obesity; they also have
a high prevalence of diabetes and I am informed that they eat much
refined carbohydrate.   Their disease patterns are totally different
from those of the Amazon Indians who live in their traditional
way and are not developing these Western diseases.   With regard to
the history of constipation, I would like to say we have found by
intestinal transit studies that people can have daily bowel actions
but very prolonged transit times.   You cannot ascertain with
certainty whether a person is constipated by asking him about the
regularity of his bowels.   Since cancer is due to an environment
that has existed for 45 years or longer, we find that you cannot
really learn accurately what bowel actions had prevailed over
previous decades.   We do not know whether patients with bowel
cancer or diverticular disease have had long transit times or low
stool weights during most of their lives.   With regard to Finland,
I would like to ask Dr. Rimpila, who is half-Finn, to comment
because he knows something about the diet in that country.

J. Rimpila: Actually, I was born in Chicago, but having lived near Finns and observed what they were eating, as well as having heard stories of what they ate in the old country, I would say that in general they use more dairy products and very little beef, intermediate amounts of pork, and other red meats. They obtain much of their protein from fish and dairy products. The fiber-content of their diet would be similar to that of populations in the U.S. and Britain.

A. Price: Could I make an observation, following Dr. Burkitt's excellent paper? If one accepts the idea that a slow transit time allows carcinogens to act over a longer period, then surely one would expect colonic cancer to be commoner than rectal cancer, for the rectum generally is believed to be empty. Rectal cancer, however, is the commonest large bowel malignancy.

N. S. Painter: I think the idea that the rectum is empty is false, and further, that the carcinogen need only be a smear on the mucosa. This is why carcinoma has a different distribution in the large bowel and rectum from that of diverticular disease, which tends to be in the sigmoid.

J. B. Kirsner: We have assumed that 70% of the carcinomas of the large bowel are located in the rectum and sigmoid area. However, someone has recently projected a change in this distribution, which would locate more of the carcinomas proximal to the rectum. Is this opinion solid?

N. S. Painter: I would not be sure.

J. Christensen: That statement was made by John Berg at the University of Iowa, who has just completed a long survey based on the records of our cancer registry, which goes back for about 50 or 60 years. It is quite clear that several decades ago the distribution was as you describe it, 70% in the rectum. That pattern now has changed so that it approximates 40% in the rectum, and the remainder more proximally in the colon.

M. M. Stanley: I would like to ask Mr. Painter about the differences in symptoms between the two groups of patients described as those with irritable colon and those with painful diverticulosis. Can one identify or separate these two groups without the aid of the radiologist or do they have the same symptoms?

N. S. Painter: I should say no; there is a big overlap. Patients with the irritable colon have more diarrhea than the others, but it is often difficult to assess.

E. V. Jensen: As an outsider to this field, I must say I found the discussions and presentations today most interesting, stimulating and worthwhile. I would like to ask three questions of Mr. Painter: You mentioned that there does not seem to be any congenital or racial influence on diverticular disease but that it seems to be mostly an enviornmental phenomenon. Is there any evidence that there is a hereditary factor? It happens that in my own family on my father's side diverticular disease is remarkably frequent. I wondered if this disorder tends to occur more often in certain families. The second question is related: Is there any way of identifying a person as a high-risk before he develops diverticular disease? In other words, can you select a high-risk group in which it might be practical to examine the prophylatic action of fiber? The third question is, in the group of patients who received bran, did you find any impairment of iron absorption? Is iron deficiency a problem?

N. S. Painter: I know of no hereditary evidence for diverticular disease of the colon. Families tend to eat as their parents do and this might be a factor. I do not know how one would isolate a high-risk group, but in a country where one in three over the age of 60 develops the disease I would say we in the Western world all seem to be at high-risk. As regards a study of the prophylactic effect of fiber; I think this should be done and I have a feeling it might work. Finally, I have noticed none of our patients becoming anemic, apart from two who bled acutely while on bran; there was no chronic bleeding and no evidence of impaired iron absorption.

K. W. Heaton: I agree that we need to initiate more studies and if I can do nothing else with what I have presented today, I hope it may have aroused enough interest to persuade others to enter what I think might be a very interesting and productive field.

D. M. Hegsted: Are there any animal models that produce diverticulosis?

G. J. Devroede: I know of two studies on animals, the rat and the dog; the rat develops diverticulosis when fed a low-residue diet and the dog does not do so. One of the major differences in structure is that the dog has a continuous longitudinal muscular layer, whereas the rat does not.

M. M. Stanley: In relation to early animal models for experimental diverticulosis, Carlson and Hoelzel (1949) of the Department of Physiology in the University of Chicago, produced diverticulosis in the proximal colon of rats by feeding low-residue diets. (See also Wierda, 1943.) Recently Hodgson (1972), using similar methods, was successful in rabbits; he did not specify the

sites of the diverticula in the colon. However, the diverticula
formations were transient and were demonstrable only after intracolonic pressure had been raised by administration of prostigmine
0.05 mg/kg. In controls not taking a low-residue diet the same
dosage of prostigmine raised pressure less and diverticula did not
appear.

A. Connell: I think it is more appropriate to call these
formations sacculations rather than diverticula. In order to
produce them the diet has to be strongly artificial. In fact, the
experimental group was grossly deficient in a number of other
features. They lost much weight as compared with the control
groups. I doubt the clinical applicability of such studies.

A. N. Smith: I should like to add that there is some doubt
as to the reproducibility of these observations. They form thick
circular muscle rather than true diverticula. The rabbits lose
weight and when I tried to repeat the Hodgson (1972) studies, the
muscle seemed to thicken by contraction rather than by a process
of true hypertrophy or hyperplasia. One of the earliest studies,
however, produced something akin to diverticula. I think in the
early 1930's Boydorr, Garry and colleagues were asked to investigate
the diet of prisoners of Peterhead Prison in Scotland. They fed
the prison diet to rats in what I think must be one of the earliest-
recorded experimental production of something similar to diverticular disease of the colon. Of course they were not really being
fed on the traditional Scottish diet for prisoners; that is porridge
and water.

G. J. Devroede: Dr. Price has said that there was some dispute
as to whether the muscle abnormality in diverticular disease was
hyperplasia or hypertrophy. Arfwidsson (1964) in his excellent
study of the subject made a mathematical analysis of this point.
The number of muscular cell nuclei per microscopic field is significantly decreased in patients with diverticular disease and cell
size is greater. So Arfwidsson concluded, and I think rightly,
that there is hypertrophy in patients with diverticular disease.

A very minor point deals with history, Dr. Smith. I am 36,
interested in history and no French nationalist; but Cruveillhier
in 1849 described the muscular hypertrophy of diverticular disease.
He also stated that the diverticula were herniations through the
muscle and then indicated that his colleague, Professor Albert
had the most diverticula he had seen. I don't know if this had
anything to do with his dietary habits. The next comment is
directed to Mr. Painter who has indicated that he did not think any
congenital factor could be involved in this situation. I agree
with him that for most patients, this is true. However, in

Marfan's syndrome, there is a higher than normal incidence of
diverticular disease at a much younger age. One of the basic
abnormalities in this syndrome is a defect in the connective tissue
of the body generally.

Finally, I have a question for Dr. Smith. His manometric data
indicate that patients who had a myotomy had a markedly increased
motility index before surgery, and this declined to a level that
was not significantly different from the control after the myotomy.
On the other hand patients who had undergone bowel resection for
diverticular disease had either inflammation and fibrosis or
muscular hypertrophy. Patients who had inflammation and fibrosis
did not have a markedly increased motility index, and they remained the same after surgery for diverticular disease with
complete resection of the rectosigmoid juntion. Every surgeon
will agree that the area where the taenae fan out to become a
continuous longitudinal layer in the rectum extends over three or
four centimeters and I wonder if this might explain some of the
results. In the myotomy operation, it has been considered crucial
to extend the incision well beyond the muscular hypertropy, above
and below. Patients with inflammation undergo resection of the
rectosigmoid junction because of edema; the surgeon has to do the
anastomosis in the normal area, well below and most likely in the
rectum. Patients who had resection and only muscular hypertrophy
are most likely to have an anastomosis that is not in the rectum,
in the area where the taenia fan out. I know of no controlled
study of this question but I would like to hear Dr. Smith's
comments on this point.

A. N. Smith: The first myotomy group consisted of patients
with obstructive features and very high pressures by which they
were selected for operation. They were compared with similar
patients treated by resection whose intracolonic pressures remained high. Patients with a fibrotic reaction after a post-
inflammatory episode also were treated by elective resection. These
patients had low intracolonic pressures which tended to remain low
after operation. In those patients in whom the pressure did not
rise, the resections were limited so perhaps some of the affected
bowel was left. We do not perform wide resections--mainly the
pelvic colon. It also is possible that resection in this group
was lower or below the alleged sphincter at the pelvi-rectal
junction. If that is removed, the patient generally is cured of
symptoms. So that probably in this resection group the pressure
remains low after resection without requiring a wide excision. The
bowel may have been damaged or we may have accomplished a more
critical reduction of intracolonic pressure by a local excision
which fortuitously has removed the most important area of the bowel
in relation to this problem.

M. H. Floch: Our epidemiologic group studying colonic disease
in Connecticut would like to thank Dr. Burkitt and the other
British scientists for stating their very stimulating theory.
Accepting the facts that there are high- and low-risk populations,
that one of the differences in the populations is the diet and that
transplantation of populations or changing their diet without transplantation of people increases the risk; we further postulated
that there may be a dietary difference among the high-risk population. The only convenient technic available to study diet-intake
variables among individuals is the diet history. We have not discussed the problems of diet history today and there is little
experience evaluating retrospective diet-analysis in disease states.
However, our epidemiologists at Yale agree with the validity of
diet history studies and we have begun to collect data from 21
subjects. We compared subjects with normal sigmoidoscopy and
barium enema to individuals with colonic carcinoma and with diverticular disease. Seven-day retrospective diet histories were done
on each subject and the total food-intake was computed from
standard food tables (Bowes & Church) for all known content,
including carbohydrate, fiber, cholesterol, fats, all amino acids,
minerals and vitamins. No differences were found among the three
groups, except surprisingly, there was significantly less fat
intake among diverticular patients than in the normal or carcinoma
subjects. Fiber-intake varied in individuals between 1.4 and 8.7 g
per day, but the mean was low in all three groups. Admittedly,
these are few cases and our diet studies will be expanded, but I
would appreciate Dr. Burkitt's comments on our initial observations
and on the variable-risk factors among high-risk populations.

D. P. Burkitt: My interpretation would be that whether or not
people in this country develop the diseases associated epidemiologically with a low-fiber diet, virtually everybody consumes such
a diet. We have genetic differences of susceptibility to environmental factors. Everybody who smokes cigarettes does not get lung
cancer. In Australia there is a high incidence of skin cancer but
everyone exposed to much sun does not develop it. Since almost
everybody in North America is on a relatively low-fiber diet it may
be just the "luck of the draw" or a genetic difference that decides
who develops a particular disease. It has been suggested by
Wynder (1967) that vegetarians probably have about a 20% lower
prevalence of bowel cancer than non-vegetarians and they have a
higher fiber diet. I think we should look at communities in a
wider context than North America to relate disease patterns to the
fiber content of diet.

J. B. Kirsner: I might comment on some studies in progress at
the College of the Medical School in Loma Linda. They have been kind
enough to send me some of their data. In their population group of
Seventh-Day Adventists there is a very definitely decreased intake

of protein and fat and a very high incidence of vegetarians. Their
data would indicate a very much lower incidence of bowel cancer as
well as a lower incidence of atherosclerotic cardiovascular disease
among Seventh-Day Adventists.

P. M. Berman: We all recognize that long-term control studies
will be necessary to determine whether dietary fiber plays a role
in either the prevention or treatment of diverticulosis. A
reference was made earlier to the paper by Monousos which described
studies of two populations in Greece, one an urban and another a
rural population, and the authors assured us that dietary intake
of both groups were the same. However, they found a much higher
incidence of diverticulosis in the urban, higher socio-economic
class than in the rural group. I wonder if Dr. Burkitt could
comment about this study and how it fits with his concept.

D. P. Burkitt: I do not know anything about this Greek study.
All I could say is that in areas we have studied in India and the
Middle East it is always members of the upper socio-economic group
who develop diverticular disease first, and we have attributed this
trend to a dietary change. Perhaps one example might illustrate
this point. In Shiraz several years ago, I was told that they had
seen only five cases of diverticular disease in eight years. One
of these was a millionaire who had built the hospital; one was a
wealthy banker; one was a landowner; one a general, and I am not
sure what profession the fifth person represented. These are
people who first are at risk of developing diverticular disease
whether or not it is due to diet.

D. M. Hegsted: I would like to comment on Dr. Floch's remarks
and to agree with Dr. Burkitt that I think we ought to look, but
I do not think we should be surprised if dietary histories do not
correlate with our current views. Certainly in relation to the
evidence on cardiovascular disease or circulating serum lipids for
this country, the genetic variable appears to be greater than the
dietary variable. Outside the United States there appear to be
some correlations that make sense but this same relationship is not
apparent within the United States. So I agree with Dr. Burkitt
that in every chronic disease there is a genetic condition upon
which the dietary variable works. For example, 30% of American
men who eat an atherogenic diet never develop an elevated serum
cholesterol; there must be genetic influence here. On the other
hand, dietary modifications do influence serum lipids in nearly
everyone.

B. Levin: It is clear that there are many factors involved in
the causation of colon cancer. With respect to a recent study by
William Haenzel and John Berg from the National Cancer Institute
and the University of Iowa on Japanese who migrated to Hawaii, it

would appear that besides the change in dietary fiber intake, they
found a significant increase in the amount of beef consumed by
these individuals. This relates to one of the current theories on
the etiology of colonic cancer, namely, a relationship with the
intake of saturated fats, particularly those contained in beef.
It also would appear that there is a high incidence of colonic
cancer in populations who consume large amounts of beef, particularly in certain parts of Scotland, New Zealand and Australia.
But in Argentina, where large amounts of beef are consumed with
large amounts of fiber (their diet is certainly not fiber-depleted),
the incidence of colonic cancer also is very high.

   D. P. Burkitt: I do not know the prevalence of bowel cancer
in Argentina. High beef diets may relate inversely to fiber content, as does sugar. It is a question of trying to determine which
dietary factor is the relevant one. If there was a constant
relationship between beef consumption and bowel cancer, then one
should be able to postulate some kind of hypothesis as to what it
is in beef that causes cancer, but I doubt whether there is any
universal correlation. There may just happen to be a correlation
in one or two places. I very much doubt whether much beef is eaten
in Scotland today in view of its price. It is, however, past and
not present experience that would be relevant.

   G. J. Devroede: The merit of Manuosos' study is to point out
that there are many variables involved in the problem of diverticulosis. Its incidence was significantly greater in the urban
than in the rural population. People in the higher socio-economic
levels had a greater incidence than those in the lower levels.
Most important and pertinent to today's discussion, there was no
difference in the incidence of diverticular disease between subjects
on a low or high intake of cellulose.

   A. F. Hofmann: May I engage in a brief speculation and try
to put together some of Dr. Burkitt's ideas with some of Dr.
Heaton's ideas and develop a logical relationship between fiber,
bile acids, gallstones, constipation and diarrhea. At the present
time we think that one of the villains in gallstones is increased
cholesterol concentration in the liver and in bile secreted by the
liver. Excess hepatic cholesterol results from a high-fat, high-
cholesterol diet and from a relative deficiency of chenodeoxycholic
acid. Dr. Heaton says that the reason this occurs is because we
eat too little fiber, and I think that that is perfectly reasonable,
although the problem needs more study.

   Obviously, the way to treat this problem is to starve, or to
take chenodeoxycholic acid, or to take more fiber. Dr. Henri
Sarles (Marseilles, France) told me that during the war in France
when they suffered severe caloric restrictions, cholelithiasis

seemed to disappear. I also think it is of interest to compare
cholestyramine, another polymer with fiber. Fiber pulls bile acids
into the colon, but here the fiber is attacked in part by bacteria,
releasing the bile acids which cause inhibition of water absorption
with an increase in fecal weight. By contrast, cholestyramine
binds bile acids tightly, and patients experience constipation.
The National Heart Institute in the United States is initiating an
extensive trial of cholestyramine for patients with type II hyper-
lipidemia. Many of these patients will develop constipation. The
question is, are they going to develop bowel disease as a consequence? So cholestyramine also causes a decrease in chenodeoxycholic acid in bile but it has its undesirable effects. The fiber
situation then becomes all the more interesting because of its
several desirable therapeutic properties.

   Dr. Storey: Several points made by Dr. Dietschy concerning
fiber and cholesterol metabolism should be further analyzed. He
indicated that rats which changed from fiber-free to fiber-containing
diets had increased rates of cholesterol synthesis. This trend would
be in accord with our theoretical mechanism of the involvement of
fiber in cholesterol metabolism. Introducing fiber into the diet
would decrease cholesterol absorption by binding cholesterol and
bile acids. This would result in lower levels of circulating
cholesterol and in increased cholesterol synthesis. Table 1
demonstrates the involvement of fiber in cholesterol metabolism
and atherosclerosis. Moore (1967) fed rabbits diets that contained
cellophane, cellulose, wheat-straw or peat as the source of fiber.
Plasma cholesterol levels are highest when the most inert type of
fiber is fed and lowest when natural types of fiber are used.

TABLE 1. Influence of Roughage on Atherosclerosis in Rabbits Fed
Cholesterol-Free Diets

Roughage	Weight Gain (kg)	Plasma Cholesterol (mg/dl) ± SEM	Degree of Atherosis ± SEM
Wheat straw	0.46	114 ± 12	12.7 ± 3.0
Cellulose	0.49	133 ± 10	20.8 ± 2.9
Cellophane	0.46	216 ± 14	37.5 ± 6.8
Cellophane-Peat (14:5)	0.47	141 ± 12	10.7 ± 2.0

   After Moore (1967). All diets contained 20% butter fat, fed
for 40 weeks.

TABLE 2. In Vitro Binding of Sodium Taurocholate by Various Substances

	% Bound ± SEM	
Substance	Experiment 1*	Experiment 2**
Cholestyramine	81.5 ± 0.2	---
Colestipol	57.0 ± 0.5	---
Cellulose	0.5 ± 0.5	---
Cellophane	0.4 ± 0.7	---
Alfalfa	16.9 ± 0.7	34.5 ± 0.2
Wheat straw	1.8 ± 0.8	---
Bran	0.7 ± 0.7	---
Oregano	---	46.3 ± 0.2
Parsley	---	40.8 ± 0.6
Sage	---	24.7 ± 1.0
Celery	---	12.7 ± 0.2
Bagasse	---	5.6 ± 0.4

*40 mg of binding substance, 100μmoles of sodium taurocholate.
**100 mg of binding substance, 100μmoles of sodium taurocholate.

TABLE 3. Influence of 1% Alfalfa in Semi-Purified Diets on Cholesterol Metabolism in Rats (3 weeks feeding)

	Dietary Group (6/Group)	
	Semi-Purified (SP)	SP + Alfalfa (1%)
Weight gain, g	65 ± 6*	62 ±
Liver weight, g	7.9 ± 0.4	9.8 ± 0.4**
Cholesterol		
Serum, mg/dl	102.7 ± 5.4	84.3 ± 6.0***
Liver, mg/100g	292 ± 20	213 ± 18
Serum plus liver pool, mg	31.3 ± 0.5	27.5 ± 1.4***
Absorption (after 0.5μCi of 4-^{14}C -cholesterol)		
Serum (dpm X 10^4)	2.69 ± 0.44	1.66 ± 0.28
Liver (dpm X 10^4)	6.03 ± 0.88	5.97 ± 0.66
Feces (dpm X 10)		
Neutral steroid	4.38	6.86
Acidic steroid	1.46	2.00
% absorption	46.9	19.5

*Standard error   **p < 0.001   ***p < 0.05

Atherosis parallels these differences. To test our theory that
fiber influences cholesterol absorption in part by binding bile
salts, we carried out experiments in which sodium taurocholate was
incubated with various types of fiber and the amount of bile salt
bound to the fiber was measured. (Table 2) Natural types of
fiber bind bile salts to a much greater extent than synthetic
types. Table 3 presents the results from an experiment in which
rats were fed semi-purified diets to which 1% alfalfa was added.
There is a drop in serum and liver cholesterol and a big difference
in cholesterol absorption as measured by fecal recovery of a
radioactively-labeled, oral dose of cholesterol. This can be
attributed in part to the ability of alfalfa to bind salts and
cholesterol resulting in a greatly reduced absorption of cholesterol. Thus fiber's involvement in cholesterol metabolism is an
important consideration.

REFERENCES

Carlson, A. J., Hoelzel, F., 1949, Relation of diet to diverticu-
     losis in rats, Gastroenterology, 12:108-115.

Hodgson, W. J. B., 1972, An interim report on the production of
     colonic diverticula in the rabbit, Gut, 13:802-804.

Moore, J. H., 1967, The effect of the type of roughage in the diet
     on plasma cholesterol and aortic sclerosis in rabbits, Brit.
     J. Nutr., 21:207-215.

Wierda, J. L., 1943, Diverticula of the colon in rats fed a high
     fiber diet, Arch. Path., 36:621.

Wynder, E. L., Shigematsu, T., 1967, Environmental factors of
     cancer of the colon and rectum, Cancer, 20:1520-1561.

PART V

SUMMARY

CONFERENCE SUMMARY

J. H. Cummings

NRC Gastroenterology Unit, Central Middlesex Hospital

London, England

If we examine the list of diseases currently thought to be due to a lack of fiber in the diet (Table 1) then the reasons for this conference are readily apparent. The list includes carcinoma of the large bowel, today probably the commonest cancer in the world, and ischemic heart disease which claims as many lives in the West as do all types of cancer combined.

EPIDEMIOLOGY

As Mr. Burkitt, Mr. Painter and others (Trowell, 1972a) have pointed out, the primary evidence linking this group of disorders with dietary fiber is based upon epidemiology. With colonic cancer as an example, there is general agreement that international differences in its incidence exist. The age-standardized incidence for the male South African Bantu is 10.5 per 100,000 population (colon and rectum) whereas the incidence in Connecticut, U.S.A., is 65.2 per 100,000 (Doll, et al., 1970). That these differences are not genetic in origin is evidenced by the comparable incidence amongst the white and Negro populations in the U.S.A. and by the rise in the incidence in Japanese who move to Hawaii (Glober, et al., 1974). Although international differences in the incidence of other diseases, such as carcinoma of the stomach, exist, the distinguishing feature of the "fiber-deficiency" disorders is that their distribution is similar, and coincides with variations in dietary fiber intake. The rural African has a mean crude-fiber intake of 24.8 g/day (Lubbe, 1971) whilst in the West crude-fiber intake is about 5.0 g/day (Robertson, 1972). The "fiber-deficient" disorders thus are prevalent in areas where fiber intake is low.

TABLE 1. Fiber-Deficiency Disorders

Colonic	Related Disorders
Constipation	Dental caries
Hemorrhoids	Obesity
Diverticular disease	Diabetes
Appendicitis	Atheroma and ischemic
Colonic polyps	heart disease
Carcinoma of colon	Venous thrombosis
	Varicose veins
Other Gastrointestinal	
Gall stones	
Irritable bowel syndrome	
Hiatus hernia	

This hypothesis may be an oversimplified view of the situation. Closer examination of the diet of the rural African (Lubbe, 1971; Lubbe & Maree, 1973) reveals that it differs in almost every respect from that eaten in the West. At an international level, dietary fat and protein intakes correlate more closely with the incidence of colonic cancer than does dietary fiber (Drasar & Irving, 1973). The prevalence of ischemic heart disease, which has been the subject of extensive epidemiological investigation, correlates also with dietary fat and in addition with cholesterol intake (Bronte-Stewart, et al., 1955; Keys, 1970). Whilst it is true that our data on dietary fiber intake in these various communities are inferior to the data for other dietary constituents (see later), these correlations with other foodstuffs require explanation. The fiber hypothesis also fails to explain the pronounced regional difference in the incidence of "fiber-deficient" disorders such as that which exists for diverticular disease in Scotland, or why people with similar fiber intakes should have different incidences of colonic cancer. Further, as Dr. Mendeloff mentioned, the incidence of appendicitis, a fiber-deficient disorder, is falling rapidly in the U.S.A., without there being any rise in fiber intake. Finally, two other epidemiological correlations have been mentioned which do not fit in; the high prevalence of ischemic heart disease in Finland in contrast to their low colonic cancer incidence, and the close correlation between the incidence of colon and breast cancer internationally (Drasar & Irving, 1973). Clearly, a revised hypothesis is necessary to explain these additional facts, which although including fiber will, as Mr. Burkitt points out, relate other environmental factors to the etiology of these disorders.

THE NATURE OF FIBER

A recurring theme throughout this meeting has been our ignor-
ance of exactly what constitutes fiber. This is partly due to the
confusing terminology used to describe fiber. Until recently the
most widely used term was just "fiber" or "crude fiber" which
refers to those substances measured by a time-honored and legally
defined procedure for the assessment of the fiber-content of
animal foodstuffs (Kent-Jones & Amos, 1967). This method measures
mainly lignin and cellulose, is empirical and underestimates the
total fiber content of a particular material by a factor of five
to ten times. Unavailable carbohydrate, a term introduced by
McCance and Lawrence in 1929, describes those carbohydrates in the
diet that are not hydrolyzed by enzymes secreted by the human
gastrointestinal tract (McCance & Lawrence, 1929). It is now
realized that this cannot be applied strictly to fiber, since it
is neither completely unavailable nor entirely carbohydrate. At
the present time the most useful term for the fiber fraction of
the diet is "dietary fiber", first used by Trowell (1972b) and
which is coming to include the whole of the constituents of the
plant cell wall resistant to the normal digestive processes of the
human small intestine (Trowell, 1974).

The problem of a clear definition of fiber is compounded by
the relative lack of satisfactory analytic data on the fiber
content of our diet (Cummings, 1973). Only two groups in the
world have made any systematic attempt to approach this question
from both the biochemical and nutritional aspect and they are
Southgate at the Dunn Nutritional Laboratories in Cambridge,
England, who is looking at this from the viewpoint of human nutrition
(Southgate, 1969) and Van Soest at Cornell University, Ithaca,
U.S.A., who leads the animal nutritionists in this respect
(Van Soest & McQueen, 1974). The reason for this lack of knowledge
is because fiber is no simple organic molecule but an extremely
complex polymeric structure. Chemically, fiber comprises four
main groups of substances: cellulose, the hemicelluloses, the
pectins, all of which are carbohydrates, and a non-carbohydrate
group, the lignins. All are large polymers, some unbranched like
cellulose, but the others are all highly branched molecules that
intertwine and encircle each other to form the complex structures
we term fiber. Chemical estimation of the amount of fiber in food
therefore is difficult, and separation of fiber into its constituent parts even more exacting.

The amount of each component of fiber present in the cell wall
varies from plant to plant (Southgate & Durnin, 1970) and so
different plant fibers can be expected to have different physiological effects. In this respect a useful distinction can be drawn
between fiber derived mainly from cereals and that of fruit and

vegetable origin. In addition, the relative amounts of lignin
present will alter the metabolism of fiber considerably (Raymond,
1969).

What is also apparent if an attempt is made to analyze fiber
is that not only is it a complex substance but it does not occur
in nature as a "pure" form. Fiber is integrally associated with a
wide variety of substances which are present in the plant cell
wall such as the metal ions: magnesium, maganese, silica, calcium
and potassium; phytic acid; fat and protein. This point is particularly relevant when one considers how often in an experimental
study of the effects of fiber the investigators are really looking
at the cereal fiber present in bran. Bran is only about 31%
dietary fiber, the rest being soluble carbohydrate (starch, sugar)
28%, protein 13%, fat 4%, moisture 13% and ash 5%. Bran is even
less of a standard preparation than fiber, and these differences
may account for apparently conflicting results from individual
experiments. There is clearly a need for more analytical data,
not only chemical but possibly some sort of biological assay for
this heterogenous group of substances.

The complexity of fiber, whilst being a problem to the analytic
chemist, is in some respects one of its main virtues. Not only is
its chemical composition important but fiber has characteristic
physical properties. Dr. Eastwood has dealt with these and their
possible implications. Four physical characteristics are of
particular importance: its capacity to take up water and swell;
its cation exchange properties; its capacity to absorb organic
molecules such as bile salts; and its gel properties. These
functions of fiber are relevant to its ability to alter fecal
weight, intestinal transit time, affect bile salt and therefore
cholesterol metabolism, and bind various ions in the gut. The
physical characteristics of fiber vary from one source to another
and what is equally important is that they are liable to be
altered or even lost when fiber is "purified" or pre-treated with
solvents prior to being used in an experimental situation. This
is particularly so when "pure" forms of fiber such as cellulose,
solka-floc and lignin are being used. In these circumstances any
effect ascribed to the treated preparation may not be seen when
it is present in its "natural" form as part of the cell wall.
Similarly, the digestibility of fiber is altered, usually reduced,
by prior treatment which alters its physical composition
(Van Soest & McQueen, 1974).

EFFECTS OF FIBER

During this conference we have focused upon those effects of
fiber which are relevant to colonic disorders. The experimental

support for the fiber hypothesis lags considerably behind the
epidemiological evidence, yet certain facts about fiber are
emerging.

There seems little doubt that adding fiber to our diet
increases fecal weight. Reports of fiber not increasing fecal
weight require closer examination but this probably can be explained by simultaneous changes in the rest of the diet balancing
the effect of fiber, or by inadequate experimental control.
Precisely how fiber increases fecal weight is not yet known
although several theories have been put forward for its mode of
action (Cummings, 1973).

When one examines the data on fiber and transit time the
picture is less clear. In general, transit time decreases as stool
weight increases (Burkitt, et al., 1972) but there are reports of
transit not changing significantly with marked changes in fecal
weight (Eastwood, et al., 1937). Where a subject has a fast
transit time before fiber is added to his diet, then fiber may slow
it down and this has led Dr. Heaton to postulate that fiber
"normalizes" colonic activity(Harvey, et al., 1937). At the
present time, our concept of transit through the gut is perhaps
an oversimplified one and our methods for measuring it are rather
crude. Movement through the gastrointestinal tract, particularly
the right colon, probably does not resemble a long column of
material travelling towards the rectum. Mixing, streaming and
turbulent flow occur, thus limiting the value of information
derived from the appearance of a fixed amount of marker or
pellets in the stool after a single bolus (Edwards & Beck, 1971;
Findlay, et al., 1974a). In the end, however, it is likely that
fiber will be shown to influence significantly the way in which
food residues pass through the gut.

The effects of fiber upon colonic motor activity relate mainly
to diverticular disease. In diverticular disease of the colon,
there is an exaggerated response of colonic intraluminal pressures
to food and to prostigmine. This response correlates with the
pathological changes seen in diverticular disease, i.e., muscular
hypertrophy. Muscular hypertrophy is thought to result from the
colon having to propel fiber-depleted, hard, small-volume stools.
Giving bran to patients with diverticular disease both lowers their
colonic pressure responses (Findlay, et al., 1974b) and as
Mr. Painter has shown, will improve the patients symptomatically
(Painter, et al., 1972). Bran, therefore, would seem to be of
therapeutic value in diverticular disease, but its role in the
prophylaxis of this condition, which is the gist of the epidemiological theory, is unproven. Mr. Smith's post-operative studies
are the first useful pointers to the prophylactic effect of fiber.
Giving bran to patients who have had surgical correction of their

diverticular disease prevents the return of the characteristic
exaggerated pressure responses post-operatively, particularly after
surgical myotomy.

The situation with regard to fiber, bile salts and lipid
metabolism is less clear. Animal experiments suggest that dietary
fiber increases fecal bile salt excretion (Portman & Murphy, 1958)
and this has been demonstrated in man (Stanley, et al., 1973;
Antonis & Bersohn, 1962). However, Dr. Eastwood was unable to
show an increase in fecal bile-salt excretion when bran or cellulose
was added to the diet of normal volunteers (Eastwood, et al.,
1937), but he has shown that dietary fiber, by increasing stool
weight dilutes the fecal bile salts. The concept of bile salt
concentration in the feces requires clarification, since bile salts
are probably not equally distributed throughout the solid and
water phases of stool. Thus, the physical state of bile salts both
in the stool and at all levels of the gut is of great importance
with reference to fiber. Dr. Heaton has presented data which show
that bran alters bile salt metabolism, not by altering overall
synthesis but by reducing the production of deoxycholic acid,
reducing the deoxycholate pool size and increasing the chenodeoxycholate pool. Overall there was no change in total pool size
(Pomare & Heaton, 1973). The implication is that whereas fiber
may not increase bile salt output, it significantly alters its
metabolism so that ultimately cholesterol synthesis falls, the
solubility of cholesterol in bile is improved and plasma triglyceride levels fall. This assumes that cholesterol synthesis is
controlled by a feedback of absorbed bile salts from the intestine,
particularly the ratio of deoxycholate to chenodeoxycholate; a
fact which Dr. Dietschy has pointed out is not proven. Reduced
synthesis of deoxycholate without a change in deoxycholate
excretion are not mutually incompatible facts as Dr. Hofmann
explained.

The work of Hill et al. (1971) on the fecal microflora from
various parts of the world showed significant differences between
areas of high- and low-fiber intake. Dr. Eastwood has reported no
difference in fecal flora of people from Scotland with fast and
slow transit time and I know of two studies in progress where
adding fiber to a controlled diet has not altered the numbers nor
the distribution of species of bacteria present in the stool. It
is possible that changes in fecal flora occur only over a very
long period, but what may change more rapidly is the metabolic
capabilities of the resident flora.

Finally, the metabolism of fiber. There is little doubt that
some fiber is broken down in the human gut by intestinal microflora, particularly the hemicellulose fraction. What then happens
to the metabolites of fiber (mainly short-chain fatty acids) is

unknown but Dr. Levitt's preliminary studies on colonic absorption
of carbohydrates suggest that the colon can absorb appreciable
quantities of carbohydrates probably in the form of short-chain
fatty acids. Fiber and its metabolites may influence normal
digestive processes as fecal fat and nitrogen excretion are increased by a high-fiber diet (Southgate & Durnin, 1970). However,
this may not represent true malabsorption, as fiber is integrally
bound to fat and protein in the plant cell wall, and the fat and
protein may not be available to normal digestive processes.

PROSPECT FOR FIBER

If it ultimately proves desirable to increase the fiber intake
in our diet, we shall be faced with the prospect of reversing an
historic trend. One of the seemingly inevitable accompaniments of
"civilization" is the removal of fiber from the diet, especially
cereal fiber. Where man has choice between the high-fiber diet
such as that of the rural African and the low-fiber, refined,
convenient types of food available to his urban counterpart, then
he chooses the latter. In Britain, despite there being a large
choice of bread, white, brown and wholemeal, available to the
housewife, only 8.3% choose brown or wholemeal bread (Flour
Advisory Board, 1974). Before we press our countrymen to change
their eating habits, there is a need for much more experimental
evidence on the effect of fiber on human physiology. The analysis
of fiber is complex but excellent biochemistry is a prerequisite
to any experimental studies. Fiber undoubtedly alters gastrointestinal function, but the evidence already suggests that the
simple "fiber hypothesis" needs modification to include the role
of other components of the diet. Controlled clinical trials of
fiber in the prophylaxis of colonic disorders are needed, as well
as further epidemiological studies focused on the regional variations in disease, and on trends in disease patterns. Extra
fiber in the diet may have undesirable effects, particularly in
terms of calcium, iron and zinc metabolism, and like any substance
if taken to excess may provoke unwanted results (McCance &
Walsham, 1948).

REFERENCES

Antonis, A. and Bersohn, I., 1962, The influence of diet on fecal
    lipids in South African White and Bantu prisoners, Am. J.
    Clin. Nutr., 11:142-155.

Bronte-Stewart, B., Keys, A., Brock, J. F., Moddie, A. D., Keys,
    M. H. and Antonis, A., 1955, Serum cholesterol, diet and
    coronary heart disease. An inter-racial study in the Cape
    Province, Lancet, ii:1103-1107.

Burkitt, D. P., Walker, A. R. P. and Painter, N. S., 1972, Effect
    of dietary fiber on stools and transit times, and its role in
    the causation of disease, Lancet, ii:1408-1412.

Cummings, J. H., 1973, Dietary fiber, Gut, 14:69-81.

Doll, R., Muir, C. and Waterhouse, J., 1970, Cancer incidence in
    five continents. International Union Against Cancer,
    Springer-Verlag, Berlin, 1970.

Drasar, B. S. and Irving, D., 1973, Environmental factors and
    cancer of the colon and breast, Brit. J. Cancer, 27:167-172.

Eastwood, M. A., Kirkpatrick, J. R., Mitchell, W. D., Bone, A. and
    Hamilton, T., 1937, Effects of dietary supplements of wheat
    bran and cellulose on feces and bowel function, Brit. Med. J.
    iv:392-394.

Edwards, D. A. W. and Beck, E. R., 1971, Fecal flow, mixing and
    consistency, Am. J. Dig., Dis., 16:706-708.

Findlay, J. M., Mitchell, W. D., Eastwood, M. A., Anderson, A. J. B.
    and Smith, A. N., 1974, Intestinal streaming patterns in
    cholerhoeic enteropathy and diverticular disease, Gut,
    15:207-212.

Findlay, J. M., Mitchell, W. D., Smith, A. N., Anderson, A. J. B.
    and Eastwood, M. A., 1974, Effects of unprocessed bran on
    colon function in normal subjects and in diverticular
    disease, Lancet, i:146-149.

Flour Advisory Bureau Press Notice, Guardian, 29th July, 1974.

Glober, G., Klein, K. L., Moore, J. O. and Abba, B. C., 1974,
    Bowel transit times in two populations experiencing similar
    colon cancer risks, Lancet, ii:80-81.

Harvey, R. F., Pomare, E. W. and Heaton, K. W., 1937, Effects of
    increased dietary fiber on intestinal transit, Lancet,
    i:1278-1288.

Hill, M. J., Crowther, J. S., Drasar, B. S., Hawksworth, G., Aries,
    F. and Williams, R. E. O., 1971, Bacteria and etiology of
    cancer of the large bowel, Lancet, i:95-100.

Kent-Jones, D. W. and Amos, A. J., 1967, Modern cereal chemistry,
    Food Trade Press, 6th Edition, p. 564.

Keys, A., 1970, Coronary heart disease in seven countries, Circu-
    lation, 41:Suppl. 1.

Lubbe, A. M., 1971, A comparative study of rural urban Vanda males
    Dietary evaluation, S. Afr. Med. J., 45:1289-1297.

Lubbe, A. M. and Maree, C. M., 1973, Dietary survey in the Mount
    Ayliff district: A preliminary report, S. Afr. Med. J.,
    47:304-307.

McCance, R. A. and Lawrence, R. D., 1929, The carbohydrate content
    of foods, Med. Res. Counc. Spec. Rep. Ser. No. 135.

McCance, R. A. and Walsham, C. M., 1948, The digestibility and
    absorption of the calories, protein, purines, fat and calcium
    in wholemeal wheaten bread, Brit. J. Nutr., 2:26-41.

Painter, N. S., Almeda, A. Z. and Colebourne, K. W., 1972, Unpro-
    cessed bran in the treatment of diverticular disease of the
    colon, Brit. Med. J., ii:137-140.

Pomare, E. W. and Heaton, K. W., 1973, Alterations of bile salt
    metabolism by dietary fiber (bran), Brit. Med. J., iv:262-264.

Portman, O. W. and Murphy, D., 1958, Excretion of bile acids and
    B-hydroxysteroid by rats, Arch. Biochem. Biophys., 76:367-376.

Raymond, W. F., 1969, The nutrition value of forage crops, In
    Advances in Agronomy, Vol. 21, (N. C. Brady, ed.) pp. 1-108,
    Academic Press, New York and London.

Robertson, J., 1972, Changes in the fiber content of the British
    diet, Nature, 238:290-292.

Southgate, D. A. T., 1969, Determination of carbohydrates in foods,
    II. Unavailable carbohydrate, J. Sci. Food Agric.,
    20:331-335.

Southgate, D. A. T. and Durnin, J. V. G. A., 1970, Caloric
    conversion factors. An experimental reassessment of the
    factors used in the calculation of the energy value of human
    diets, Brit. J. Nutr., 24:517-535.

Stanley, M. M., Paul, D., Gacke, D. and Murphy, J., 1973, Effects
    of cholestyramine, Metamucil and cellulose on fecal bile
    salt excretion in man, Gastroenterology, 65:889-894.

Trowell, H., 1972a, Ischemic heart disease and dietary fiber, Am.
    J. Clin. Nutr., 25:926-932.

Trowell, H., 1972b, Crude fiber, dietary fiber and atherosclerosis, Atherosclerosis, 16:138-140.

Trowell, H., 1974, Definitions of fiber, Lancet, 1:503 (Letter).

Van Soest, P. S. and McQueen, R. W., 1974, The chemistry and estimation of fiber, Proc. Nutr. Soc., 32:123-130.

APPENDIX

FIBER CONTENT OF WHEAT AND WHEAT BASED FOODS

This conference included a presentation on the chemical methods used to determine food fiber and the need for more exact information on chemical composition. Since grain, particularly wheat, is usually considered the most important dietary source of fiber in the American diet, some description of the wheat grain and resulting fiber content of finished food products appear appropriate.

Recent studies (Food and Nutrition Board, Nat. Acad. Sci. U.S.A., 1974) have shown that about 26% of the daily calorie intake of the U.S. population comes from food products based on cereal grains. However, this amounts to 17% on a flour equivalent basis. This paper will include a brief review of the wheat grain, source and location of fiber in wheat as well as fiber content of finished foods.

Several excellent reviews of wheat grain structures and composition are available (Pameranz and McMasters, 1968; Bradbury, et al., 1956; Toepper, et al., 1972). These include anatomy and nutrient distribution throughout the wheat kernel. Additionally, the Wheat Flour Institute has prepared an excellent schematic diagram of how wheat flour is milled.

The wheat kernel may be divided into three major components (Wheat Flour Institute). The endosperm, from which white flour is made, amounts to about 83% of the kernel. Bran, a constituent of whole wheat flour and breakfast cereals, represents approximately 14.5% of the wheat grain, and wheat germ which is also usually separated in flour milling is about 2.5% of the wheat kernel. The latter is also frequently used in breakfast cereals as a means of adding protein.

TABLE 1.   Fiber and Starch Levels of Wheat Milling Fractions

Wheat Fraction	Percent Fiber	Percent Starch
Wheat	1.7-2.6	54.1-61.8
Flour	---	64.3-73.7
Wheat germ	2.8-4.0	14.0-23.9
Bran	9.2-11.6	4.6-7.2

Composition of Foods, U.S.D.A., 1963
(from Pameranz and MacMasters, 1968)

The bran portion of wheat grain is made of the outer cell
layers including the seed coat, spidermis, hypodermis and
aleurone cells. The amount of endosperm adhering to this outer
coat or bran will vary depending on milling practices.

The typical range of fiber and starch levels in these milled
wheat fractions are shown in Table 1.

Food products containing whole wheat flour, wheat germ and
wheat bran contribute dietary fiber in varying levels, whereas
those containing white flour contain practically no fiber.

TABLE 2.   Fiber and Total Carbohydrate Content of Wheat Flours and
Foods

Food	Percent Fiber	Percent Total Carbohydrates
All purpose wheat flour (enriched & unenriched)	0.3	76.1
Cake or pastry flour	0.2	79.4
Whole wheat flour	2.3	71.0
Shredded Wheat Breakfast Cereal	2.3	79.9
40% Bran Flakes Breakfast Cereal (Kellog Co.)	3.5	76.4
Bran breakfast cereals (Kellog Co.)	7.0	68.1
Enriched white breads	0.2	50.4
Whole wheat bread	1.6	47.7

Composition of Foods, U.S.D.A., 1963

The actual fiber and total carbohydrate levels in wheat flours and wheat based foods are shown in Table 2.

Although the total, or average, dietary intake on a per capita basis is unknown, the above data provide information that may be useful in designing high-fiber diets.

REFERENCES

Bradbury, D., Cull, I. M. and MacMasters, M. M., 1956, Structure of the mature wheat kernel, I. Gross anatomy and relationship of parts, Cereal Chemistry, 33:329.

Composition of Foods, 1963, Agriculture Handbook No. 8 U.S.D.A., Washington, D.C.

Food and Nutrition Board National Academy of Sciences, 1974, Proposed Fortification Policy for Cereal-Grain Products, Washington, D.C.

Kellog Company, Battle Creek, Michigan 49016.

Pameranz, Y. and MacMasters, 1968, Structure and composition of the wheat kernel, Bakers Digest, XLII:24.

Toepper, E. W., Palansky, M. M., Eheart, J. F., Slover, H. I. and Morris, E. R., 1972, Nutrient composition of selected wheats and wheat products, Cereal Chemistry, 49:173-186.

Wheat Flour Institute, 309 W. Jackson Blvd., Chicago, Illinois 60606.

PARTICIPANTS

Thomas P. Almy, M.D.
Dartmouth Medical School
Hanover, New Hampshire

Denis P. Burkitt
Medical Research Council
London, England

James Christensen, M.D.
Department of Internal Medicine
University Hospital
Iowa City

Alastair M. Connell, M.D.
Gastric Laboratory
Cincinnati General Hospital

J. H. Cummings, M.D.
M.R.C. Gastroenterology Unit
Central Middlesex Hospital
London, England

G. J. Devroede, M.D.
Faculte De Medicine
University De Sherbrooke
Sherbrooke, P.Q., Canada

John M. Dietschy, M.D.
5323 Harry Hines Boulevard
Dallas, Texas

M. A. Eastwood, M.D.
Department of Clinical Surgery
Western General Hospital
Edinburgh, Scotland

B. H. Ershoff, Ph.D.
Institute for Nutritional
  Studies
Culver City, California

Martin H. Floch, M.D.
Norwalk Hospital
Norwalk, Connecticut

Sherwood L. Gorbach, M.D.
Chief, Infectious Diseases
Veterans Administration Hospital
Sepulveda, California

Kenneth W. Heaton, M.D.
Bristol Royal Infirmary
Bristol, England

D. Mark Hegsted, M.D.
Harvard University Public Health
Department of Nutrition
Boston

Alan F. Hofmann, M.D.
The Mayo Clinic
Rochester, Minnesota

John H. Hopper, Vice President
Food and Drug Research
The Kellogg Company
Battle Creek, Michigan

Elwood V. Jensen, Ph.D.
Department of Physiology
University of Chicago

Joseph B. Kirsner, M.D., Ph.D.
Louis Block Professor of Medicine
University of Chicago

Albert C. Kolbye, Jr.
Dir. Off. of Sciences-Bur. of Foods
HEW-Food & Drug Admin.
Washington, D.C.

Louis E. Kovacs, President
Vitamins, Incorporated
Chicago

Rueven Levitan, M.D.
4325 Grove Street
Skokie, Illinois

Michael D. Levitt, M.D.
178 Malcolm S.E.
Minneapolis, Minnesota

A. I. Mendeloff, M.D.
Sinai Hospital
Baltimore

N. S. Painter, M.S., FRCS, FACS
Manor House Hospital
London, England

Sydney F. Phillips, M.D.
The Mayo Clinic
Rochester, Minnesota

Ashley Price, M.D.
Pathology Department
St. Mark's Hospital
London, England

Richard W. Reilly, M.D.
Department of Medicine
University of Chicago

Irwin H. Rosenberg, M.D.
Department of Medicine
University of Chicago

Marvin M. Schuster, M.D.
Baltimore City Hospitals
Baltimore

Adam N. Smith, M.D.
Gastrointestinal Unit
Western General Hospital
Edinburgh, Scotland

Howard M. Spiro, M.D.
333 Cedar Street
New Haven, Connecticut

Malcolm M. Stanley, M.D.
318 Southcote Road
Riverside, Illinois

Philip L. White, Sc.D.
American Medical Association
Chicago

Ifor P. Williams, M.D.
Northwick Park Hospital
Harrow, England

Charles S. Winans, M.D.
Department of Medicine
University of Chicago

Robert W. Wissler, M.D., Ph.D.
Department of Pathology
University of Chicago

SUBJECT INDEX

Absorption, from human colon, 51-65

    at various levels, 56
chemical modifications of, 58
electrolyte, 56
measurement of, 61-65
physical modification of, 59

Alfalfa, effect on cholesterol metabolism in rats, 160

Almy's law, 95

Atherosclerosis, in rabbits, and roughage, 159

Available carbohydrate, 4, 6

Bile salts

    bacterial degradation of, 27
interrelations with fiber and bacteria, 17-20
production, as affected by diet, 41

Bran

    as normalizer of colonic activity, 86
bleeding after consumption of, 153
prophylactic role in diverticulosis unproved, 169

Bran, commercial, in Great Britain, 41

Bran, effects of

    after surgical operations on colon, 131-133
cholesterol in bile, 34
fecal bile acids, 30, 33